Praise for This Book

It has been an honor to witness the love, strength, and unwavering commitment that shaped this story of Sally and John's journey through dementia. However, this book is more than a journey through that disease. It is a testament to devotion, resilience, and the power of standing beside someone you love through life's most difficult chapters. With honesty and grace, John opens a window into the realities of caregiving, heartbreak, hope, and enduring connection. Anyone who has walked this path, or may one day, will find comfort, understanding, and profound humanity in these pages.

I had the honor of visiting with sweet Sally frequently. We laughed, cried, and shared how much God loves us. She always had a Bible sitting on the dining room table, along with a devotional book of some kind. Her commitment to her Christian faith was a witness to all. Thank you, John, for your honesty and for allowing us to walk with you during this journey. My prayer is that this book will help others understand the path their loved ones may be on and how to navigate each change that will take place.

—CHARLOTTE MCCONNELL

When I started our Men's Golf Bible Study about 15 years ago, I needed help from someone who was trusted and experienced in ministry. John fit the bill. As a local pastor and an avid golfer, he was known as someone who "practiced what he preached." His golf balls had a distinct logo on them, allowing people to know that he was a Christian. During the studies, we often talked about how to treat our wives, and everyone knew that John deeply loved Sally.

When Sally was diagnosed with her condition, people from within the Bible study, as well as those outside, watched to see how he handled the challenge. Would he blame God or abandon Sally? It was a resounding "No" to both questions.

John showed us how to navigate this difficult challenge. He now has a platform to talk from experience when he meets people going through something similar. As you read this book, you'll see the devastating progression of dementia/Alzheimer's in Sally. However, I believe you will discover hope, encouragement, and peace if someone you care about is facing this illness.

—DICK MORTON

God blessed me with far more than a neighbor's cup of sugar when He brought sweet Sally into my life. From the moment we moved to Huntsville, TX, she welcomed me with open arms, sharing her love for Jesus, stories from her colorful life, and that radiant bridal joy that always lit up her smile. She became my dearest friend—we shared coffee and long, peaceful walks nearly every day.

Watching John care for Sally through this final chapter of their abundant marriage was the most beautiful dance of devoted, unconditional love I have ever seen. In the midst of heartbreaking loss as our Sally slowly slipped away, his bravery, endless patience, and tender care revealed a grace only God could weave—even through the sorrow. This book gently shares their story to prepare others for what may lie ahead, offering hope and understanding in the journey.

—CONNIE GRISHAM

GLIMPSES

My Wife's Journey Through
Dementia and Alzheimer's

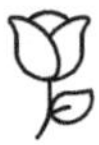

John Burchell

HARVEST CREEK PUBLISHING AND DESIGN

This book is a work of non-fiction. Every effort has been made to ensure that all the information on these pages was accurate at the time of publication.

The views expressed in this work are solely those of the author and do not necessarily reflect the views of the publisher.

Scriptures marked as "NLT" are taken from the *Holy Bible*, New Living Translation, copyright © 1996, 2004, 2015 by Tyndale House Foundation. Used by permission of Tyndale House Publishers, Inc., Carol Stream, Illinois 60188. All rights reserved.

Scriptures marked as "RSV" are taken from the Revised Standard Version of the Bible, copyright © 1946, 1952, and 1971, the Division of Christian Education of the National Council of the Churches of Christ in the United States of America. Used by permission. All rights reserved.

Scriptures marked as "NKJV" are taken from the New King James Version®. Copyright © 1982 by Thomas Nelson. Used by permission. All rights reserved.

Book Cover & Interior Layout © 2026 Harvest Creek Publishing & Design

Harvest Creek Publishing & Design
www.harvestcreek.net

GLIMPSES—1st ed.

ISBN 978-1-961941-51-8

Printed in the United States of America

Contents

Dedication

To my Sally,

My Baby, my companion for 50 years,
the one who always made me smile.

Rest in peace, my love.

Acknowledgements

Currently, I am still able and blessed to continue serving the two churches I have been leading for over 14 years. They have walked with me and helped pick me up when I needed them, particularly over the past few years of Sally's life. They saw her decline and stepped in to help in ways that really can't be explained. One would have to experience what I went through to fully understand what these two congregations did for me.

Handwritten cards were sent, telling me they were with me and would always be there for me during this horrific journey. The Christian love that was given unconditionally to me was truly what I leaned on to help get through the days spent dealing with this disease that ultimately took Sally's life. I knew the path would be difficult, but the journey was longer and more painful than I had ever experienced before.

During the first six months following her graduation from this life to the eternal life was like a fog. My normal daily schedule continued, such as leading the Bible study for the people of Focused Care every Tuesday morning. There were so many rewarding times with all those residents who would faithfully attend those services. And I felt closer to Sally by being with them.

The staff at Focused Care were wonderful to work with. They provided excellent care for Sally before her graduation. Their knowledge and emotional support helped the family make the important decisions that were needed for my wife's end-of-life care.

The Men's Bible Study continued in my subdivision, early on Tuesday mornings, before the study at Focused Care. They encouraged me and helped me through some of my roughest times.

Day-to-day contacts continued with the many people we had known in Huntsville. These friends stuck with me during this time of grief by meeting me periodically for lunch or other activities. The days rolled by, and I kept reasonably busy but not so busy that I was overwhelmed. I tried to keep things simple and somewhat organized. When an event was scheduled on a particular day of the week, it gave me something to look forward to. But I was still just going through the motions. Our friends provided comfort, peace, and support during these most difficult times, especially as I was learning to walk this new path in life without my Sally.

Foreword

As a fellow United Methodist pastor, I have known John and Sally Burchell for over twenty years. I first met John through the meetings we had as pastors in the North District of the United Methodist Church. John and Sally lived in a nearby town just south of Texarkana, Texas. They were a good team in ministry. John loved people, and so did Sally. Sally was also involved in a women's organization called Celebration Women's Ministry and helped my wife as they ministered to women who desired a deeper walk with the Lord.

Besides being in ministry together, we also shared a love of golf. In fact, John and Sally were responsible for my wife, Cindy, taking up the game. One weekend, I was going to join John and Sally for a game of golf, and my sweet wife said she would like to tag along and play with us, even though she had no clubs. Sally graciously shared her clubs with Cindy. We had a great time together, and by the time Cindy got to the fourth hole, she said to me, "This is going to cost you more than this game." That afternoon, Cindy and I went out and bought a set of clubs. From that day, John, Sally, Cindy, and I often got together and played golf. We were blessed with a deepening friendship.

What struck me most about John and Sally was their deep love for each other. Theirs was a relationship where faith and love were mutually shared over many years together. They were also good golfers. I knew I had to behave when playing golf with John and Sally. They were an inspirational team, not only in golf but in life, and in the way they cared about people.

As time went by, Cindy and I moved from Texarkana, as did John and Sally. We could not play golf and get together, but later I was able to see

John regularly through a clergy small group in the Brazos Valley area. (We are still meeting today.) During that time, Sally was struggling with serious dementia. John faithfully cared for her at home, but reached a point where he had to put her in a care facility.

His visits to her were constant. And along the way of loving Sally, John developed a ministry to the people in that care facility. It was moving to hear John talk about it.

John decided to write *Glimpses*—a book fully dedicated to Sally—and I believe you'll find it as encouraging and uplifting as I have. Sally's life was so consistent in sharing unconditional love. John and Sally certainly *are* a good team, even though Sally is in heaven awaiting her beloved husband.

REV. GARRY MASTERSON
Pastor, United Methodist Church,
Author of the devotional series, *Got Wisdom?*

Preface

The Celebration of Life service for Sally ended, and everyone departed at approximately 1:00 p.m. The entire family headed across the street to the General Store for the dinner that had been prepared for us. When we arrived, Laura came and asked if we were ready to eat. We were ready, so the family gathered around, joined hands, and offered a prayer thanking our Lord for the day. I asked the Lord to please bless the food and be with everyone who would be traveling home, getting them home safely.

We served ourselves and sat down to eat. Linda, one of the church members leading the others in serving us, informed me that the two churches I serve had gotten with Jerry, the owner of the General Store, and were covering the cost of the meal. Another unexpected blessing! After the meal, there was some leftover grilled chicken breast, so those who wanted them were given take-home boxes for their trip.

At 3:30 p.m., we left the restaurant. Johnna and Tonya were with me, so I was blessed to make the one-hour trip home to Huntsville with my daughters! They talked about the service and the number of people who were in attendance. I told them both that it has been my experience throughout my ministry that how a person impacts people and their lives is directly related to the number and variety of people who attend their Celebration of Life service. We had people attending who ranged in age from their early twenties to their nineties. Sally affected everyone she met during her life.

We went to the house and had a pleasant evening just being together before Tonya had to leave the next day to go back to her family and home. Then Johnna was heading home on Monday. Both could attend church service with me on Sunday. What a day! Getting to preach two times in two days to both of my wonderful daughters. Come Tuesday, I would be home, completely alone.

Tuesday arrived. Everyone had left and arrived back home safely. I was now left in the home my late wife and I purchased together in 2012. All the paperwork had been executed, and everything had been financially resolved. This house that Sally and I turned into a home filled with love was now mine, and I was home alone. It has been a little over one month since Sally left and made the journey with the angels and Jesus to receive her mansion in the Father's house.

Throughout our marriage, we were constantly together, no matter what either of us enjoyed doing. With few exceptions, we did everything together. We both invested time and effort in learning each other's hobbies to stay close. For example, Sally enjoyed bowling, which I had never done. My favorite pastime was hunting, which she had never done. To say the least, our love for each other inspired each of us to change. We changed so that we could spend more time together while also enjoying the newly learned activity.

Until the onset of dementia/Alzheimer's, our life together was very fulfilling. Even after the diagnosis, we did everything we could to spend as much time as possible together. There was nothing more enjoyable than being with her, watching and hearing her laugh, and getting to see her glorious smile. Her brother once said of Sally's smile, "It took over her face to the point where there was nothing left but her smile."

My position as the ultimate caregiver and advocate for my wife was not unique. Spouses are often placed in this position, and they do what I did—everything possible to make sure their loved one has what is needed for a quality life. This does not mean that those placed in this position do not go through times of deep pain. But for me, as Sally's caregiver, blessings came regularly beyond belief, which gave me tremendous hope.

Sally is physically gone and missed by all who knew her, but let me tell you, she is still a significant part of my life and my thoughts. I find myself making decisions based on the way we made decisions in our marriage. It feels like she is still here with me. After over fifty years of being one together, there will never be a time when she is not part of me in my thoughts and actions.

What do I do now? What am I feeling? What will this new life be like now that I am alone? Challenging but fulfilling—with memories, thankfulness, and faith as my close companions.

The continued *Glimpses* of her in my life and my personal faith give me hope that we will be together once again. Until then, I can live each day in peace, because of this expectant hope, because of my faith, and because she told me it would be so!

Introduction

This writing is coming from a man (that's me!) who has gone through a difficult experience in his life with the wife he loved and cherished for just over fifty years. During those fifty years, our marriage was based on togetherness, love, and tremendous joy. The reason for writing this was to share some of the time spent with her *before* this disease called dementia/Alzheimer's entered her brain. And then contrast that with the challenges we faced together *during* her journey with this disease.

After reading this book, hopefully you will have a better understanding of how this disease affects the person and impacts the family. Included in shaded boxes is current information about dementia/Alzheimer's and some strategies that helped me get through difficult times.

Hopefully, everyone who reads this book sees that, *because* of this disease, the closeness to my wife *increased* more than I ever thought possible. Not only were there glimpses periodically of Sally and who she was before this disease took over, but when the disease reached its later stages, blessings from her *continued*. Her beautiful soul bubbled up and spilled out to those around her in ways I had never even known possible before the disease took over her life.

A description of her early life in Wichita, Kansas, from childhood to adulthood, will focus on the experiences that made her a strong woman. One such experience involved the marriage to her first husband, Bobby Armstrong, and his untimely, unexpected death. One beautiful result of their marriage was the birth of two loving children: Johnna and Kenny.

The situation that surrounded our first introduction was God-ordained. We were brought together by several people who thought the world of her (not totally sure what they saw in me), but they knew her well and wanted her to be happy again. I will share more about that experience, how our love sprouted and grew at a rapid pace, and from my perspective, why it happened the way it did. You will learn about a woman who had faith in her Lord and Savior, who was strong and unwavering, something I had never experienced so profoundly with anyone before.

Anytime a couple faces a difficult time in their marriage, like an unwanted medical diagnosis, their true love and unification will be tested. Hopefully, you, the reader, will see how we felt about and dealt with the issues that came before us during this journey to the end of this disease, which took her life. Alzheimer's progressed and eventually took control of her mental capabilities for most of a twenty-four-hour day. However, daily glimpses of the wife she once was still surfaced, clear in her behavior, expressions, and speech. These are referred to as *"glimpses"* throughout the book.

The unfortunate reality of this disease is that, currently, the medical community has no actual answers for an Alzheimer's cure. They have no way to stop it or slow the progression. However, everyone who is exposed to this disease, including the caregivers, the family, and those diagnosed with it, can come together to give each other a glimmer of hope. Through deep faith, we can trust that no matter what the outcome will be, our Lord is in control and has ordained every day of our lives before we were ever born into this world.

Perhaps from my experience, you, the reader, will see that even when life takes tough turns, there is still hope. Through a connection with the Lord, and that connection extending through to the one you love, you can also witness glimpses of the one you love. They will still be there.

They will be as close to you as they always were. Your loved one will still bless you beyond belief.

The key is to be ready, no matter what turn life takes, to receive those images of the one you love. Begin every day with the desire to see and be with the one you love, and let them remain a part of you and your life.

JOHN BURCHELL

ONE

The Early Years

---

*We were created for the purpose of giving God's
invisible character a glimpse of visibility.*

BETH MOORE

It was Monday, September 16, 1940, in Wichita, Kansas. That was the day that my beautiful Sally was born to her father and mother, Wilfred and Marjorie Smith. She was their first child together, but Marjorie had a four-year-old son, John, from her previous marriage. Sally's birth was uneventful, and everything went well with no problems. She had everything a child born in 1940 was supposed to have, and was welcomed and loved by her parents and older brother.

Sally grew up in Wichita with her mother, father, and brother while living on South Classen Street in the home of her grandfather and grandmother. It was during World War II, so things were precarious throughout the United States. The military draft system had been put into place to fulfill the needs of the military. Sally's father, Wilfred, better known as "Willie," was exempt from the draft and military service because of his age and the fact that he was married with two children. Willie was a truck driver and hauled live cattle to the stockyards on the north side of Wichita, Kansas. His job was steady and provided a financial means, about average or maybe a little below average, for that time in Wichita.

Sally and her family were active in Saint Mark's Episcopal Church. Her grandpa, John Thomson, was one of several architects who designed that church, which made Sally very proud. While growing up in Christian service, her faith became very meaningful to her. Faith in God the Father, Jesus the Son, and the Holy Spirit became the core of her being.

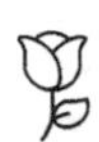 **Glimpse:** A lifestyle and way of living, according to the commands of the Bible, were always exhibited in the way she lived and treated others, no matter who they were.

During Sally's childhood, she went through normal ups and downs, including the diseases of chickenpox, measles, mumps, the flu, and so on. While attending the Wichita public school system, she was an above-average student. She carried a "B" average throughout her public-school career and graduated from Wichita High School East in May 1957. After graduation, she did not continue her education and did not attend a college or university. She did what was very normal and common for young ladies of that time—she fell in love and married.

SALLY WAS INTRODUCED to her first husband, Bobby Armstrong, by some friends, and after a period of dating, he proposed. She accepted his offer of marriage, and Sally and Bobby Armstrong began their life as husband and wife.

Bob, as he was referred to, was an auto mechanic. He opened his own repair shop with an emphasis on high-performance modifications and racing. He and Sally became partners in an auto repair shop named Armstrong's Dyno. Bob was well known in the Wichita area for his abilities as a person who could get everything out of a car's engine that was possible. He had a large following of drag racers who raced at the local drag strip.

Their business grew, and Bob branched out into building racing engines for some of the local drag racers and dirt track racers. Bob stood behind his engines. If you had a problem, Bob would come to your location and fix the problem you were having.

Not only was their business growing, but Sally became pregnant and gave birth to their first child, a boy, Kenny, in 1959. Just about two years later, she gave birth to her second child, a girl, Johnna, in 1961. Her doctor warned Sally about having any more children, even though she would have liked more. There was an RH blood factor between her and Bob. In the early sixties, this RH blood factor was very serious, and thus, the doctor's warning.

As Armstrong's Dyno Shop expanded, more engines were made for more racers, and Bob, a racer himself, spent Sundays at local racetracks. For Sally, this interrupted her time in worship at her church. For most, this would have caused their faith to diminish, but not Sally. She found ways to continue to worship and to grow her faith, even though she might not be at Saint Mark's Episcopal every Sunday.

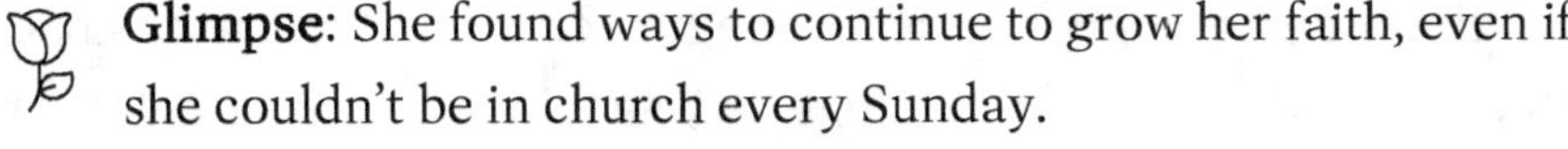 **Glimpse:** She found ways to continue to grow her faith, even if she couldn't be in church every Sunday.

TWO

Life Takes an Unexpected Turn

Grief is the price we pay for love.
Queen Elizabeth II

Every year at the Kansas State Fair held in Hutchinson, Kansas, dirt track races were held. These races attracted a rather large number of racers, probably because the purses (the amount of money you could win) were very large. Before the racing ever started, those who had entered could come to the track and practice or run "hot laps" to test and tune their car.

Bob had built a new engine for one racer, and he was experiencing some performance issues coming out of the turns. He contacted Bob and told him of the issue. He was given some things to check and told to call back. The hope was that one of the things he was told to check would fix the problem. But if not, Bob would come to them.

The items that Bob recommended him to check did not have any effect on the performance of the engine. So, Bob loaded up in the Armstrong's Dyno truck and headed to Hutchinson to fix the problem. When he arrived, he went right to work, checking everything and making sure the adjustments to the engine were correct. The problem with the car, as it was explained to Bob, was that everything was fine until the driver went to full throttle coming out of turn two or turn four. That was when the engine had a definite stumbling or hesitation.

The car was readied to go and sent out onto the track for testing. Bob went to the inside of turn two in the infield, so he could listen to the engine as it accelerated out of turn two. When the car came by, he could hear what was happening, and he had them bring the car in for an adjustment. Bob made a slight adjustment to the carburetor float height and sent the car back out onto the track.

He took his position in the infield just past the exit of turn two, the same place he had stood before. When the car came out of the turn, and full throttle was applied by the driver, the engine roared with no further hesitation. The problem was fixed.

Before they had time to celebrate, two other cars in the corner bumped into each other, and the car on the inside came down through the infield. By the time the driver saw Bob, he could do nothing with the car to avoid hitting him. The car ran right over Bob, and when it did, it crushed part of his head. The track medical people were there instantly. They loaded him into the ambulance and transported him to the local hospital.

He was placed in the medical ICU, and life support systems were connected to him to maintain his life. Sally was called, and after grabbing a close friend, she was on her way to the hospital in Hutchinson, not knowing what she would find when she arrived.

I can only imagine what was going through her mind concerning the condition of her husband. She had experienced times before when Bob was hurt because of a racing accident, so she was not dealing with something new. One thing I am sure of is that she was praying during the trip, which was less than one hour.

Upon arrival at the hospital, she and her friend went right to the ICU, where the doctor in charge met them. They went and sat down in the consultation room. He immediately told her he had some bad news concerning Bob. He proceeded to tell her the details of his injury. He also told her that the only reason he was breathing and his heart was beating was because of the life support systems. The doctor told her he had virtually no detectable brain activity.

This news hit her very hard. She was a young woman of 32, with two young children, who owned a business where she only knew the bookkeeping end. She broke down, and she cried, oh, how she cried. Her friend, Joyce, helped her through this disastrous time, but Sally responded relatively quickly.

Glimpse: She decided she was going to be all right because of her strong faith.

She called for the doctor, he returned, and she asked if she would have to decide to disconnect the life support, and if so, when?

The doctor explained that since they had detected, although very faint, some brain activity, nothing would be done until the third day. The doctor also told her she would not have to decide to unplug the life support. When no brain activity was found, he would disconnect the life support. So now all she could do was pray and wait.

During this time, she contacted her children and explained the situation concerning their father. Since both were young, she did not think they really understood, but she was staying at the hospital, and their grandmother would be at home with them.

Those two days went by slowly, but finally the third day came. The doctor arrived at the ICU and told her he was headed to check on Bob and see where he was concerning brain activity. The doctor went about his evaluation, which just took a few minutes. A couple of close friends came to the hospital that morning and were there with her, waiting for the news from the doctor. He finally finished his tests, and he turned to her and told her that her husband had absolutely no brain activity. He was gone.

Sally mourned painfully and experienced the type of pain that only a person who has been through this type of loss can understand. She continued to pray, and she felt like her Lord had his arms around her and was holding her. After what seemed to be a short time to some, she picked herself up and went back to work. She took control of her life and that of her children, as well as her business. She did things that no one thought she could do. But they did not know how strong a woman she was and how deep her belief was that her Lord would see her through this time. As she always said, "I'm going to be all right!"

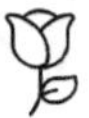 **Glimpse**: Because of her deep belief in the Lord, she always said, "I'm going to be all right!"

THREE

John Comes on the Scene

*If life can remove someone you never
dreamed of losing, it can replace them with
someone you never dreamed of having.*
RACHEL WOLCHIN

Meet a man named John (that's me) who had known Sally and Bob for several years. At that time, I was the factory territory manager for the Champion Spark Plug Company and serviced about one-third of the state of Kansas. My home base was in Wichita. My first wife and I had divorced, and we had one child, a girl (Tonya), who was three years old.

The store that Sally and Bob owned, Armstrong's Dyno, was one of my customers. Bob often talked with me concerning the use of Champion spark plugs. He was not a big fan of the Champion brand because most of his business was with General Motors and their products.

Bob had introduced me to his wife, Sally. She was there every time I called on this business.

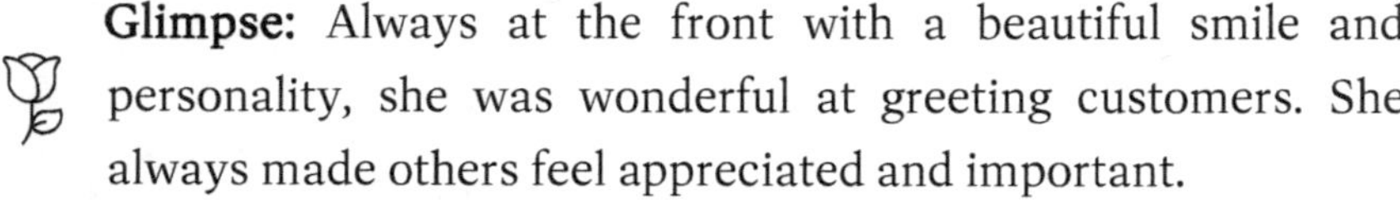

Glimpse: Always at the front with a beautiful smile and personality, she was wonderful at greeting customers. She always made others feel appreciated and important.

She knew that part of my marketing strategy included free promotional items. She would always smile and say, "Hello, John. What did you bring me today?" Most of the free items were usable—pens, notepads, coffee cups, mugs, and the like. While they were meant for advertising, she acted like they were a huge deal. That was her personality.

MY TRIPS TO Armstrong's Dyno went on even with her husband gone. On my visits, I attempted to reassure her, "Hello, Sally. Please let me continue to help you in any way possible. Whatever your business needs, let me know."

She had some Champion spark plugs in stock that were not being used. "Thank you, John. Could we possibly get credit for some spark plugs we aren't using? If not, can they be exchanged for some we could use?"

After taking an inventory of the spark plugs in question, I offered to exchange them for ones they used regularly. She was fine with that. "Here's your receipt. One of my distributors should be able to make the exchange."

IN THE AUTO repair industry, especially the independent shops, most owners knew many of the other owners, especially if they were in the same type of business. So, in Wichita, most of the shops that fell in performance enhancement and racing knew each other. It was a pretty close-knit group, particularly with a few of the better shops, and they helped one another when possible.

All those shops knew of the tragedy that happened to Bob. And they saw how strong Sally was and what a sharp businesswoman she had become. She could not fix a car, but she did well overseeing the business, and the customers enjoyed dealing with her.

Another part of my job was to keep the independent shops up to date with information from the various automobile manufacturers. I supplied them with up-to-date technical information from the various manufacturers, like Ford, General Motors, and Chrysler. This was a great help in their attempts to repair certain issues with a particular automobile if they had the manufacturer's information or technical bulletins.

From time to time, a local shop would allow me to set up a display and work the drive, talking to customers who were there for gasoline about getting their cars' spark plugs changed. The shop would receive a special price on my spark plugs, so they in turn could offer their customers a discount on changing their spark plugs. These marketing efforts helped the people doing auto repair, so hopefully they would consider and use my brand of spark plug.

One day after working the drive at a rather large service station (that was what they were called in the early 70s), I went inside to visit Ted, the owner of Ted's Dyno. After checking the inventory of spark plugs, the order was made.

Ted greeted me. "Hi, John. Joyce is in the office." Joyce took care of the financial books for their business. After checking the inventory, a replacement order was made with Joyce.

She asked, "John, would you like a cup of coffee? Ted's on his way over here."

"Yes, thank you, Joyce."

Then she surprised me with the next question. "Are you dating anyone?"

"No, nothing serious. I've been on a couple of dates, but that's all."

She continued to press for more information. "How do you feel about older women?"

Where was she going with this?

Ted walked in during my answer, "I have no problem with older women." He laughed, and we joked about it. Ted rarely laughed at work.

Joyce finally got to the point and suggested, "Sally Armstrong would be a lot of fun."

"Well, I knew her husband, Bob, so it probably wouldn't work."

THE FOLLOWING DAY, after packing the company car, I headed out west towards Greensburg and checked into the local hotel. Jack, who had a motorcycle/lawn mower/chainsaw store, did a lot of small engine repairs. He had invited me to come and visit anytime. We usually ordered something to eat and worked together on repairing some of his customers' equipment. That evening we repaired a bunch of chainsaws and a few lawn mowers.

Then Jack asked me, "Are you dating anyone of interest?"

"No, there is no one regular in my life. In fact, I'm not looking for that type of relationship right now."

"You should consider taking Sally out. She would be a lot of fun." *There it was again.*

After getting over my shock, I came back at him with the question, "Why don't you take her out?"

"Can't. I was friends with her husband, Bob."

"Same here. We were friends." Apparently, we both fell into the same arena when it came to her.

THE NEXT MORNING, I was up early and on the road to Dodge City. On the way, I took a detour to visit a farmer whose stationary engine had needed repairs in the past. It was important for irrigating his fields. The engine kept fouling spark plugs, causing it to develop a miss and lose power, which was needed to pump the volume of water to drive the irrigation nozzles. The farmer was out by the problem engine.

"Is everything working?"

He just smiled and said, "You and your spark plugs fixed it."

"Do you need any more?"

"Absolutely!" He gave me an order that could be easily filled and sent to him from Dodge City.

After arriving in Dodge City, it was still early in the morning, but the auto parts store where my farmer buddy bought his spark plugs was open. After checking their inventory and placing his order, along with getting an order from them, I called it in to the distributor they used. The day was going very well.

Calls were then made to the repair shops in the area, and the pleasant day continued. After checking into the local hotel and unpacking my clothes, I headed for the last stop of the day and then dinner.

Jim's Automotive and Parts store was in Dodge City, where there was a very well-run and managed dirt track, which was very busy on the weekends. Jim catered to most of the racers that used that track and supplied them with their racing needs, which included my favorite spark plugs.

"Hi, Jim. Anything unusual going on? Or is everything normal?"

Jim, who had a dry sense of humor, responded, "Everything is normal, whatever normal is today!"

His inventory looked fine. He had just received his weekly order from the distributor, so there was plenty of stock. Jim usually closed his store at about 6:00 p.m., and then we would take off and go to the local steakhouse for dinner. Since he was a very good customer, my largest in Dodge City, I would pick up the tab for dinner.

While we were eating dinner, he caught me up on all the local racing events and who had been the big winners. He had a new racer who was doing well.

"Would you be willing for me to supply him with his spark plugs?" he asked.

"Sure. Here's a voucher for up to eight sets. And here are some decals for anyone who needs them or wants them."

Our conversation then became much more casual, and Jim asked, "Are you dating anyone consistently?"

"No. It's hard since travel takes up so much of my time. Being gone four nights a week doesn't seem to work out well for a relationship."

"Have you ever considered dating Sally?"

Now, this was the third person in three different cities who had asked about the possibility of me dating Sally!

"No. Since I knew her husband, it just doesn't seem right."

"Well, I think she would be a lot of fun." We finished our evening and headed in for the night.

That night in the hotel room, the questions about dating, a bit out of the norm, would not leave my mind. Three different people had brought up dating Sally Armstrong. (At this time in my life, I knew who God, Jesus, and the Holy Spirit were, but had no personal relationship with them. Praying usually consisted of giving thanks before meals. Was God trying to speak to me?)

With paperwork finished, the working trip back to Wichita from Dodge City was planned for the next day. Except for a few calls on Friday morning and mailing the weekly report, work would be finished for the week.

DURING THE TWO-and-a-half-hour drive back to Wichita, the three conversations concerning Sally wouldn't leave my mind. When my week on Friday was finished, I would try to call her.

Friday morning, the sales paperwork and expense report were ready to be mailed. From my apartment, I called Armstrong's Dyno.

"Hello. Is Sally there?"

"Yes, she is. May I help you?"

"Hi, Kenny. Would you please ask your mom not to leave? I will be there in about twenty minutes."

Twenty minutes later, she was found in the back bay washing her car. That day I was wearing a pair of dark green slacks, a green and white striped shirt, and white shoes. I was decked out for the time! When she saw me, she had a hose with water coming out. Sensing she was thinking about spraying me, my instinct was to stay back a little from where she was cleaning her car.

"Hi! I was the one who spoke with Kenny about twenty minutes ago."

"Well, since he didn't know who was calling, I almost left," she said.

"Would you like to go to Doc's and grab a glass of iced tea?"

She responded, "That would be nice."

Glimpse: It would become obvious over time that "That would be nice" was one of her favorite replies.

When we arrived at Doc's, we were seated in a booth along the front windows. Since it was the middle of the afternoon, there was only one other person in the diner besides us. We ordered our tea, and it seemed to me that she was a little nervous or something, but then I was a little nervous myself.

Our tea was delivered. "Would you like anything else?" asked the waitress.

"No, thank you. We are fine with the tea," I replied. And then it happened. She knocked over her glass of tea, and it headed right for me. I hopped out of the booth in time to miss getting soaked with her spilled tea. The server saw me jump up with the tea flowing everywhere. She came with a towel, cleaned it up, and brought Sally another glass. It was obvious Sally was nervous and embarrassed, but I encouraged her not to worry—all was well.

During the rest of the conversation, which was very casual, we talked about many things, and it was a very pleasant time. The three people who had recommended that I ask her out knew what a pleasure it would be.

The inner beauty and strength of this woman sitting in the booth at Doc's with me was amazing.

Finally, I asked her if she would like to watch the USAC midgets at the 81 Speedway that night. She hesitated for a couple of seconds, and then she said, "That would be nice."

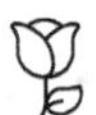 Glimpse: There it was again: "That would be nice."

SHE GAVE ME her address and directions to her home. After arriving at 6:30 p.m. sharp, she asked me to come in and introduced me to her mother, who was staying with her, her daughter, Johnna, and her son, Kenny. We then left for the races.

Thirty minutes later, we arrived at the "81 Speedway." After buying two tickets, we went in and found ourselves a place in the grandstand just at the end of the front straightaway and before the first corner. There were a few cars on the track. She held my arm firmly when they passed by where we were seated. Even though it had been well over one year since Bob's accident, that had not occurred to me when I asked if she wanted to go to the USAC midget races.

When all the cars took their places on the track, the drivers were introduced, and the engines started. Again, she held my arm firmly; again, I missed the sign. The cars started around the track, and then after they had made one full lap, the pace car exited the track, and the race was about to start. When the green flag dropped, and the cars came from the starting line headed for the first corner, Sally not only squeezed my arm, she hid her face in my side. That was when it came to me that this was bringing back the memory of the accident that killed her husband.

Immediately, we got up from our seats and left the racetrack.

"Please forgive me. I was not thinking. You are having to relive a nightmare."

She smiled, a smile I enjoyed over the next fifty years, and we left the racetrack and went to a movie theater on the west side of town. We had a very good time, and after the movie, we went and grabbed a light meal and spent time just talking.

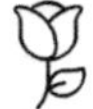 **Glimpse:** She smiled a smile I enjoyed for over fifty years.

It became clear then why she had paused before agreeing to a date.

"I'm so sorry about what happened," she said. "I thought it was something I could handle, but I was mistaken."

When we finished eating, we went to her home, and she was concerned about some cars parked out front.

"Would you like me to come in with you?"

"Yes, please." When we went in, there were two men there who had been at the racetrack. She was very upset that her mother had let them inside the house, but they promptly left. She apologized to me for what had happened.

She went on to say, "Mother, don't ever let anyone in the house at this time of night for any reason!"

On my way out of the house, I said, "I had a wonderful evening and hope we can do it again sometime."

To which she said, "That would be nice. Call me."

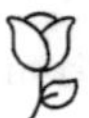 **Glimpse:** "That would be nice."

FOUR

The Start of Something Lasting: John and Sally Together

---

*Only people who are capable of loving strongly can
also suffer great sorrow.
But this same necessity of loving heals them.*

LEO TOLSTOY

Over the next few weeks, we went on a date when I was in town and not traveling. My work routine would find me leaving Wichita on Tuesday morning and returning late Thursday afternoon. On Monday and Friday, work was in Wichita. Monday was a full day. Friday, I would work until about noon and then finish up the sales report and expense report to be mailed to the home office.

We would usually see each other on Monday evening for dinner. When I was out in my territory working during the week, we would visit on the phone. Then on Thursday afternoon, after returning home, we would usually plan something very casual together.

Friday evenings, we started a tradition of getting together with her two children and grilling hamburgers. Kenny, her son, usually helped me, or rather stood around and asked questions, in place of actually helping; too many cooks spoil the meal! Sally and her daughter, Johnna, fixed French fries, baked beans, and sometimes potato salad. We then sat down at the table and ate. Kenny, a growing teenage boy, devoured the food, and thirty minutes later, he wanted something else to munch on. Then, we'd typically watch TV, and around nine, I'd say goodnight and head back to my place.

Our mutual attraction was becoming stronger every time we were together. When we were apart, we did not want to be away from each other. This pattern continued for a few weeks.

A FEW WEEKS later, Sally and her children planned a trip to New Hampshire to visit her brother, John, and his family. She and her brother were close and stayed in constant contact with each other. The brother-sister bond was very strong, and it remained that way their entire lifetimes. While happy for her and her children to get to make this trip, it was going to be difficult not seeing her for those two weeks.

The day came for her to make the trip, and she was very nervous about flying from Wichita to Boston. This would be her first time on an airplane. She was not sure what to expect.

"It will be a fun trip. You will enjoy the plane ride!" My words didn't seem to encourage her much; she wasn't buying what I was trying to sell her.

They left on a Monday morning. Two dozen long-stemmed red roses were delivered to her home right before they left.

The card read, "We have only been together for a short time, but your beauty overshadows that of these roses. Love, John." She told me later that she almost didn't go because of what the note on the flowers said.

That same day, I left for my territory and planned on spending the entire week away. Swinging out to the furthest part of the western edge, right up to the Colorado state line, my trip would be all-encompassing.

On Monday night, she called. "Hi! We made it to John's house! He has a special vacation planned for us. He's reserved a cabin in the mountains for the next ten days."

This was not good news for me because that meant no phone service and no contact with her. (This was in 1973, long before any such thing as a cellphone.) For the first time, we would be apart for two weeks. I was not looking forward to that.

Those two weeks felt like an eternity to me. During that time, I did a lot of thinking and soul-searching concerning the two of us. Where was this relationship heading? Feelings never before felt were surfacing. All kinds of emotions, all very fulfilling, were bombarding me. I was just not 100% sure of what was happening.

Looking back, it was clearly a true love event. I started looking forward to the day that she had told me she and the kids would be home, and was counting off the days!

SALLY AND HER kids returned from the trip to New Hampshire right on time. Her family had already planned to pick them up at the Wichita airport. Since I was working in town, hopefully, a message would be left at my apartment telling me she was home.

According to her, the very minute she walked into her home, she put down her luggage, went right to her phone, called me, and left a message on my recorder. It was a couple of hours before I finished my day, making calls and selling spark plugs.

Upon arriving home, the recorder was beeping, letting me know there were messages. Yes, there were multiple messages from Sally. She seemed worried about me not being home. A lot of negative thoughts had occupied her thoughts—you see, she was a real worrier. She worried about everything. Since she had been gone for a day or two over the planned two weeks, I can only imagine what she was thinking.

She must have been sitting on the phone because when I called, it never rang. She answered with an eager, "Hello!" A joyous conversation ensued.

"What are you doing for dinner tonight? Would you like to come over?"

"Absolutely!"

"Can you make it at about 5:30 p.m.?"

"Sure!"

That evening, Sally met me in the driveway just as I was getting out of the car. She grabbed hold of me as no one had ever done before. She was obviously thrilled to see me, but no more than I was to see her. It seemed this evening was one of those evenings people only dreamed of having. All those thoughts I had been experiencing while she was gone concerning where this was going were answered that night.

We picked up our relationship right where we left off before her trip. Well, that is not exactly true! For me, and for her, we were both experiencing things we were not initially expecting to happen. Lots of conversations between us took place. The type of conversations that only happened when two people were truly in love. Discussions about family, money, where we would live, how the kids would respond to me, and many, many more.

We grew closer than I had ever experienced with any person, especially closer than my first wife, Pat. During the conversations, no matter what the issue, situation, or circumstance, we always worked out our solutions for each of them, no matter what!

It WAS THE first day of July, and she was doing her monthly books and reporting to her accountant. Monthly reporting was always a stressful time for her because she did not like doing those reports, even though she was very good and exact in her computation, right to the penny! That night, she was having a real problem balancing the report, and the money just was not right. She was getting very upset and nervous.

"What's wrong?"

"I'm over six hundred dollars short." That was a lot of money in 1973, at least to us it was.

"If you don't mind, let me take a look. Maybe something will show up if another set of eyes reviews it." A few minutes later, "It looks like there aren't any credit card invoices recorded."

In those days, Mastercard, Visa, and Discover cards were not very prevalent. Instead, the norm was the oil company credit card, and this was what was not listed. We looked and found the credit card invoices. When we entered them, the report balanced right to the penny. She was so happy!

So I took advantage of the moment.

"Would you marry me?" It stunned her. She was caught off guard by the proposal.

But she looked at me, her eyes sparkled, and she answered with a resounding "YES!"

She immediately started asking me questions.

"When would be a good time of year to have it? And where should we have the ceremony? At my church or outside? How many people do you think we should invite?"

She was great at asking what I lovingly called her "twenty questions."

"It's totally up to you."

She went right to work and called the priest at St. Mark's Episcopal Church about the wedding.

"Hello, Father. I would like to request a date for a church wedding. And my fiancé and I would like you to marry us! We have been seeing each other for several months, and he has just proposed!"

"Congratulations! Tell me a little about him. Is he Episcopalian?"

"No, he's not."

"Has he ever been divorced?"

"Yes, years ago."

"Then we need him to bring all of his court documents from the divorce and meet with the bishop to get approval. But we can go ahead and set a tentative date for the wedding. The church is available on September 28. Would that work?"

"Yes! That sounds wonderful!"

In the meantime, the meeting with the bishop proceeded, and everything was approved. Sally went about organizing everything, something she was great at doing. No detail eluded her attention.

Glimpse: Sally was very organized and enjoyed taking charge of the details.

All was set, and we planned to get the invitations printed after my work trip to western Kansas. When I arrived in Dodge City and checked into the hotel, the owner's wife told me to call Sally. It was an emergency!

Not knowing what might have happened, I went to my room and called. Sally answered the phone.

"What's wrong? The hotel owner said to call you immediately—that there was an emergency!"

Evidently, the priest had called her and told her he had resigned from the church and could not marry us on our chosen date. She was beside herself and scared that our wedding would not happen.

"Don't worry!" I reassured her. "We will get together tomorrow and figure something out. We've figured out other things that have popped up, and we will figure this out, too!"

My sister, Martha, called me and told me she had talked to Sally and that she was very upset over the incident that occurred with the priest.

"Hi, John. Sally is so upset! She is afraid you might back out of the wedding! But I have an idea!" She knew how badly Sally wanted to get married in the church, but that would not happen because of the current events with the priest. She went on to tell me it would be almost impossible to find another church on such short notice.

As an alternative, she suggested we go to the county courthouse, schedule an appointment with the local judge, and go there to get married. It would not be the same as the church, but at this short notice, it would be an option. She was willing to call and find a date, but it could not be September 28 because that was on a Saturday, and the courthouse and the judge's office were closed on weekends.

Immediately, I made a call to the judge's office, and the clerk checked his calendar. He had an available time slot at 3:00 p.m. on September 23 to perform the ceremony in his office. He was leaving on vacation for two weeks, starting on the 24th. I booked the slot and was told what paperwork we would need to bring. We were set if Sally approved.

AFTER RETURNING TO Wichita, I went to see Sally and give her the news of what had been done in setting up the wedding ceremony at the courthouse. She looked at me, her eyes lit up, and she shed a few tears of excitement and happiness.

Her mother was planning to come to our wedding, which was originally scheduled for the 28th, and then she would stay there with the kids while we went on our honeymoon. When she talked to her mother, what seemed to be a normal conversation concerning our wedding made a surprising turn. She became upset that we would not be married in the church. So, she told Sally that she could not watch the kids while we were gone.

Sally was very upset at this development and was not happy with her mother. She called me very upset.

"John, my mother will not watch the kids since we aren't getting married in the church! What are we going to do?"

"Let me make a quick call. There's someone who might be able to help us."

My Aunt Waunetta was home and picked up the phone. "Hello, Aunt Waunetta. I am calling about an issue that has come up regarding my wedding with Sally. We need a sitter for the kids while we are on our honeymoon. Her mom is not available. Do you think you could help us?"

She replied, "No problem! We have plenty of room. You can bring them to me, and they can stay with us at our house. We will make sure they get to school."

"Thank you so much!" *What a relief!* "Let me call Sally and give her the good news!" A few minutes later, after speaking with Sally, her worried mind was put at ease.

Our discussion turned to Armstrong's Dyno and what the future of it looked like. Sally did not have any interest in trying to continue to operate the Dyno shop, and I did not want to give up my job as a factory representative.

She went to her key employee and talked to him about the shop. He was interested in buying the business, inventory, equipment, and various small tools. Between the two of them, they came up with what they both felt was a fair price that was good for both. Sally would keep the building and the property, and "Beav" (as they called him) would pay her a monthly rent with the option of purchasing the property at a later date.

The week before the 23rd—our new date to be married—she met with the new owner and attorneys, and the paperwork was completed. The money for all the inventory, equipment, and tools, the first month's rent, and a one-year lease were all processed that same day. Sally was relieved to get the business, which had been a struggle for her, sold, and the money deposited in the bank.

THE WAIT FOR September 23 to arrive seemed like a long time off in the future, but the days turned into weeks, and suddenly it was the 22nd. The next day, we were to go to the courthouse with Martha and her husband, Norm, as our witnesses (best man and bridesmaid). The service went well, with a few light moments.

When we went into the judge's chambers, he had all the paperwork in front of him. He looked up and smiled, stood as we shook hands, and then he said, "I am not about to ruin a perfectly good relationship, am I?"

We answered, "No!" and we all had a little laugh.

When he was administering the vows, he would barely finish, and Sally started repeating the vow. She had them memorized and was quick to respond. On the other hand, I waited until he finished, then repeated my vows. We were pronounced husband and wife at approximately 4:00 p.m. on September 23, 1974. We thanked the judge, all after the big kiss, and left the courthouse. Then we headed off to a nice club in downtown Wichita for a celebration cocktail.

Our first night together was spent at home with the kids. We packed the car and hooked up the boat. We were ready to leave for the Ozarks and our honeymoon week in a rustic cabin. We left Wichita after saying our goodbyes to the kids and making sure my aunt was ready for them that afternoon. We took the kids' clothes and other necessities to my aunt's house, and after a few moments of unloading their things, we were finally off.

THE TRIP TO our cabin on the Lake of the Ozarks went well, and after stopping for lunch, we finished the drive. We arrived at the resort and checked in with no issues. We went to our cabin and unloaded our things. Then we headed down to the marina to see if there was a boat slip we could rent while we were there. They had one available, so we rented it and found out where it was in the marina. Then we unloaded the boat into the lake, and I took it around to our rented slip and tied the boat up securely. Sally brought the car and trailer around to the marina. We decided to go out and get something to eat. Then we went to a grocery store and got a few things to eat for the week.

We had a wonderful time together on our trip to the Ozarks, and Sally did a great job helping me with the fish as they were caught. She was not a person who had ever fished much at all during her life, but she was right there with me in the boat, and she particularly enjoyed the beauty of the lake.

On our second full day, we went sightseeing, and then we returned to our cabin and fixed the fish we had caught the day before. When we returned to the cabin, I started preparing the fish and cooking dinner for us that evening. She said she was not used to having anyone fix dinner for her until now, but she loved it!

The fish tasted delicious—fresh-caught fish is always a treat—and then we went outside on the front deck and sat on a loveseat together while we watched the sunset. It seemed like the week went by extremely fast, and the day came for us to return to Wichita, pick up the kids, and get ready for the next week. The first week of our new lives together was complete.

ONCE WE SETTLED into our new life and the routines established around my work schedule, most evenings at home were spent in our den area talking and deciding what direction our lives would take going forward. She shared how much fun she had while being in the boat, watching me fish and catch a few.

She wanted to learn how to use a rod and reel so she could try to catch a fish. Her desire to learn to fish from the boat was a surprise to me, but then she was different. We would spend many moments in our boat fishing together, catching many, many fish over the years.

It came time for me to go back to western Kansas and work my territory. She indicated that her mother was in town and could come to our house and watch the kids. She wanted to go with me on my trip out west to call on customers and to make a few new ones.

"Are you sure you want to come? It may be a little boring for you."

"I don't care as long as we are together."

This type of togetherness in all things ultimately led to a very fulfilling life together. We left for western Kansas on Monday afternoon for our first working trip.

FIVE

Becoming One in All Things

We are alive in all our layers of self and
selflessness—individuals becoming one.

JAY WOODMAN

One of the big things in her life was bowling. She was a part of three different women's leagues on three different teams. Now she could work more on her bowling because she no longer had the business to be concerned with since the sale. She started practicing more, and her game improved tremendously. During her Thursday afternoon league, I would come to the bowling alley and watch her bowl. I enjoyed being there and admired her ability on the lanes.

At this time, I did not bowl and had never bowled. But learning this game was important so that we could take part in it together. Sally was excited that I was taking an interest in what she enjoyed and knew this would be a wonderful learning experience.

My brother-in-law was an excellent bowler and had shot a perfect game of 300 in a tournament once. I asked him how to go about learning this game and getting instruction on the basics, to prevent developing bad habits from the start. They're always harder to fix than they are to prevent, if one uses the right instructors.

Norm told me we needed to contact another friend who was a very knowledgeable bowler, and he could get me on the right track. So I contacted Dwayne, told him my plans, and he agreed to help me. We arranged times during the week, normally on Monday and Friday, to get together to teach me how to bowl.

I picked up the basics quickly, going to a bowling alley to practice as much as possible. Eventually, my skills improved enough to go bowling with Sally, although that did not matter to her. The fact that I wanted to be involved in what she enjoyed meant the world to her. What was novel was having someone who cared about what *she* was doing.

As my bowling skills improved, Martha and Norm, along with Sally, decided we needed to join a mixed couples league and bowl as a team. Sally was all for it, so we decided we would do just that. They found a new league that was starting on Sunday evenings at 6:00 p.m., so we joined. This league would finish by 8:30 p.m., so it seemed to be a perfect match, plus most of the bowlers were just starting in the sport. We needed, or wanted, a sponsor—some company that would buy us shirts with the company's name on the back. The spark plug company I worked for gave me a small advertising allowance, so we became the "Spark Plugs."

THE SUNDAY NIGHT bowling league ended around the end of May, so fishing was next on the list to do together. Remember me talking about how, on our honeymoon, Sally would sit in the boat as I fished? Well, she wanted to learn to cast with a rod and reel like mine. I felt comfortable teaching her how to cast with that type of equipment, so we went to work. She was a little nervous, and she said she did not want to mess up and disappoint me.

"That will never happen," I assured her.

She had some problems with the bait-casting reel, so I purchased her a closed-face reel. She handled that one with ease. We were now set to take a fishing trip and let her try out her newly learned techniques.

We planned a trip to Lake Livingston, just a few miles east of Huntsville, Texas. It was a new lake, just completed and flooded some four years earlier. The fishing there was great, but this is an enormous lake, so I found a fishing guide who would take us fishing. We loaded up early in June, left the kids with her mother, and we were off for a week of fishing.

When we arrived at the lake, we found Ray, the guide, and planned to meet him for breakfast early the next morning. We met him at the restaurant at the marina complex at 5:30 a.m. the next day. During breakfast, he asked if we wanted to go fish for black bass or if we just wanted to catch a bunch of fish. I spoke up and told him we wanted to catch a bunch of fish. The white bass were working up in the far north end of the lake, in the river and creeks that fed into the lake. We drove to a launching ramp Ray knew and used, put the boat in the water, and off we went. The excitement of this trip was more than enough for her, and we were doing it together.

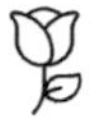 **Glimpse:** Sally found joy in all our joint pursuits, readily taking on new hobbies to deepen our time spent together.

We decided to only keep about 30 white bass, then we would quit and head back to the marina and clean the fish. Ray had a real sense of humor, and we were catching a fish on literally every cast. Most were small, but the action was great. After an hour or so, Sally was worn out from catching all those fish. She laid her rod down and just sat there in the boat seat, resting. Ray looked at her and told her, "You can't catch fish with your lure in the boat!" She picked up her rod and reel and went back to fishing.

That night, she told me that now she understood why I was so tired after fishing all day, especially after catching a bunch of fish. We showered at the shower facility at the campground, and we went to bed about 8:30 p.m. Both of us went right to sleep. I can't speak for Sally, but I believe I remained fairly still throughout the night until the 5:30 a.m. alarm the following morning.

Ray had given me directions to some places along the river and in the lake that we could access easily, and we would catch plenty of fish, which we did. Each day, we grew closer to one another.

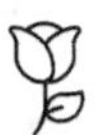 **Glimpse:** I learned from Sally the true meaning of love and how it was supposed to work.

As I've shared our story thus far, I hope you're catching *glimpses* of our shared growth, both in life and love, as we grew to become one.

THE NEXT DAY, we took the boat, and we headed out to try our hand at finding those fish along the river area of the lake. The river that was the major source of water in Lake Livingston was the Trinity River. This river, as it wound its way through the lake, had dead trees on one side of it. Ray had given me an area on the river to fish, and across from the area were three homes built on a spot that overlooked the river and the lake. We found this location with no problem. According to the fish locator on our boat, the trees were in about 10 feet of water, and then it dropped off to about 30 feet of water in the river itself.

Right along these trees, facing the river, the locator indicated a bunch of fish. As soon as we started casting, we caught fish—mostly small ones, but we caught some nice white bass. Sally was using her closed-face reel. Fighting the fish with this rod and reel was a much tougher task than I was having with my baitcasting rod and reel. She asked if she could try one of my rods with the baitcasting reel. I picked one up and tightened the drag down where she would not get a backlash, but it also limited the distance she could throw her lure.

With each cast, she was relaxing and becoming better and better. Gradually, I loosened the drag a little more at a time, which gave her more and more distance. Through her perseverance, she was learning to cast with no backlash, commonly called a "birds-nest," or "professional overrun."

She was having a great time catching these fish with her new rod and reel combination. The way she was learning to cast the lure out into the river area and bring it back to where the fish were, I could not have been prouder of her. Now I had a permanent fishing partner, and our life together was wonderful and blessed.

We made several trips to various lakes in Texas. We talked about possibly moving somewhere in Texas where we would be closer to the lakes because we enjoyed fishing so much. Kenny was out of high school and working, but Johnna was going to be a sophomore the next school year. We needed to discuss some options with her.

AFTER SEVERAL MORE fishing trips to East Texas, we decided to move there permanently. But Kenny did not want to go with us. He wanted to stay in Wichita and live with his Grandma Armstrong. However, Johnna seemed eager to go to Texas. We made a trip to Tyler to look for a house where I had also received an excellent job offer.

Sally made a remark to me that the only thing she did not like about Texas was that there were so few trees. She was thinking more about the places in West Texas she had visited during bowling tournament trips. Even though she had seen the trees around the lakes in East Texas, she was not aware that all of East Texas had similar terrain, which seemed to amaze her.

When we met with the realtor in Tyler, we discussed the size of the house we were looking for and whether we wanted to live in town or just outside. We looked at each other and said simultaneously, "Outside of town." We viewed several houses and found one that was about six miles east of town on old Highway 64. With a size of around 2500 square feet, the house included three bedrooms, two bathrooms, and a two-car garage on three-quarters of an acre of land! This house was significantly bigger than our Wichita home, and we eagerly anticipated the move.

We returned to Wichita and informed our families of our impending move. Our home was on the market. I needed to be in Tyler to start my new job in a little over one month, so we were hoping our home in Wichita would sell quickly.

Our prayers were answered, and the home in Wichita sold quickly. The movers came on the appointed day, loaded up all of our furniture, clothes, and other stuff, and we were told it would arrive the next Saturday in Tyler. We then set off for Tyler, TX, to close on our new home.

AFTER CLOSING ON Friday, we took possession of our new home, and the movers arrived on Saturday as planned. Everything was unloaded and placed in the rooms where we instructed the movers to put them, and then we started unpacking. I worked on getting our bedroom set up first, then Johnna's bedroom, while Sally and Johnna were in the kitchen working together, getting it organized.

At one point, I went out to the kitchen, which was about three times the size of the one we had in Wichita, with a really nice dining area as part of the kitchen. Sally and Johnna were sitting on the floor, and Sally was crying. "What's wrong?" I asked her.

She was overwhelmed by the size of the cabinet room; the size was daunting to her. We laughed, hugged each other, and I kissed her. They went back to setting up the kitchen after I told her she did not have to use all the cabinets right now; we would fill them later.

The next day, I went to work at my new job as the service manager of the local Lincoln-Mercury Honda dealership located in Tyler. Things were very different overseeing the service department but with my training as a factory representative, it all fell into place with only a few hiccups.

Sally wanted to help financially. She always aspired to be a part of our lives, no matter what, and she found employment at the local Sears. She went to work in the area that administered and sold maintenance agreements for appliances that people bought through Sears.

With the income from my job as service manager of the dealership, and her income from Sears, we were doing well financially. We started saving money in a savings account immediately with the plan of getting with a financial advisor once we had saved $10,000. We had money from the sale of our home in Wichita, and we had only used what was needed for the down payment on our new home in Tyler. We were doing well.

There was a nice, large bowling alley in Tyler, so we went about finding leagues we could become a part of and resume our bowling. Sally landed on two women's teams, and I found a men's team that needed a member, and we also found a couple's league that we joined. So, it seemed like we were at the bowling alley four evenings a week, and we were enjoying our new city of residence.

On the weekends, we took the boat out and fished either Lake Palestine or the two Lake Tylers. Outside of the time we were both at work, we were together. Sally had to work at Sears every third Saturday until noon, so I would take her to work and run errands until it was time to pick her up from work. Johnna was doing well in school and had taken a part-time server job at the local diner just about a mile from our house. When she finished work in the evenings, about 8:00 p.m., one of the other workers would bring her home. It seemed like things were going well.

THE ONE IMPORTANT area missing in Sally's life was her ability to do religious activities, which she desperately missed. At this time, I was still not much into that sort of thing. While I knew about God, Jesus, and the Holy Spirit, they were not a real priority in my life.

Sally met a lady, Mary Snell, who was part of the local Methodist Church. She invited Sally to go with her on Sunday mornings to their worship service. It was not the Episcopal Church, but the service in the Methodist church was very close to what she was used to, so it became her church.

I would attend church with her from time to time, but not regularly. This was the one thing, for some reason, I had no interest in getting involved in. She was thrilled on those Sundays we attended together. She would have liked me to be there every Sunday, but she was happy whenever I came.

Our bowling continued, and Sally became one of the leading bowlers in the city of Tyler. For several years, she had the highest average of all the lady bowlers in that city. People always wanted her to go with them as a team member to various tournaments. She was able to attend many of them each year and could manage her schedule at work to take a day off here and a day there to make those tournaments.

Sometimes I would travel to them, leaving Tyler on Friday evening after closing at the dealership. I would arrive at the hotel where she and the other members of the team were staying to be with her during the tournament on Saturday and Sunday. After the tournament ended on Sunday, we would travel home together.

IN TYLER, I met several men who all hunted mostly deer, but a lot of dove and quail as well. They invited me to go on a couple of dove hunts, which brought back memories about how much I loved doing that as a younger man.

Around age 12, my uncle Bob started taking me hunting with him. He would take me dove, quail, and pheasant hunting. He taught me gun safety and how to shoot. With his teaching, I became a pretty fair shot with my little 410 single-shot shotgun.

Hunting was officially added to my life, and I ultimately started hunting whitetail deer with the two men I had met. I had never hunted deer, so they had to teach me what to do and how to do it. Thankfully, I picked it up quickly, and it became a regular part of my outdoor life.

Sally was interested, but shooting a rifle in a caliber that sufficed for harvesting a deer was a little scary to her. We went out to a field and set up a place to shoot that was close to our home in Tyler. She practiced using a 22-caliber rifle with a scope, so she would be comfortable shooting a rifle with a scope mounted on it. We talked about the rifle and the dangers of rifles once we pulled the trigger.

"We have to be sure of *what* we're shooting at before we squeeze the trigger," I told her. "Once the bullet leaves the barrel, we cannot bring it back. We have to be completely sure of our target before that happens."

Women who are not afraid to shoot a gun, shotgun, or rifle tend to be better shots than men. Sally had no problem with a shotgun, so this 22-caliber rifle was a breeze for her, and she was very accurate. I told her how proud I was of her and her shooting ability, which brought the smile I loved so much.

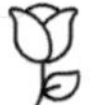 **Glimpse:** She had a big, beautiful, joyful smile!

We continued to hunt doves and quail. Sally used one of my shotguns. She was an accurate shot, and one evening after a few days of hunting, she said she would like to get her own shotgun. She had talked to Seth, a man we hunted with on a lease. He had a nice 20-gauge shotgun that he did not use anymore. He had purchased it after he had had shoulder surgery because the recoil, "kick," was less, and he could use it without doing any damage to his surgically repaired shoulder. I suggested that if she was comfortable with that shotgun, I would support her in the purchase of it.

She took the shotgun and practiced with it multiple times. She used it on a pheasant hunt that all of us took part in, which was held on a game ranch. She did well with the shotgun, so she and Seth worked out the price and a short payment plan, and the purchase was made. She was happy with her new shotgun. She had come a long way as a hunter, and I told her so!

When deer season came around, we made plans to take a vacation. We wanted to hunt the second week of the season at our lease in Uvalde with Seth and his wife. Sally asked me what rifle she was going to use on this hunt.

"You should have your own rifle," I told her. "It could be your Christmas present from me."

The next day, we went to the local gun dealer in Tyler and asked him what caliber he would recommend for her. He recommended a .243 caliber because it was more than enough for harvesting whitetail deer, yet it had a light recoil. He gave her several brands of rifles to hold and to shoulder as if she were going to shoot.

Sally decided on her favorite, but the gun dealer needed to shorten the stock so the rifle would fit her better. She chose a scope, and the dealer said everything would be ready the next afternoon, around 5:00 p.m.

We went together to pick up her new rifle the next afternoon, and it was ready. She sat down in a chair with a rest built on it, and she looked through the scope while the store owner made sure it was properly mounted for her. After a minor adjustment, he took it to the back of his store and fired the rifle to make sure it was shooting where he aimed. We paid for the rifle and headed to our spot where we practiced shooting.

We placed the target about 100 yards away, and she sat in the shooting seat with a rest and prepared to fire her first round from her new rifle. She took her time, and then she squeezed the trigger. The bullet hit the target about two inches high and about two inches to the right of the bullseye. I made a quick scope adjustment for her to correct the sight to zero. She took her rifle, took her time, and fired the second shot, and hit the top of the bullseye. We celebrated her accuracy, and she fired a few more times just to get used to the rifle. She was fast becoming an excellent shot with her new rifle.

Friday night, at about 9:00 p.m., we arrived at the lease. Seth was already there. We grabbed a bite to eat, discussed which stands we would hunt the next morning, and went off to bed. Our day started with an early rise at 5:30 a.m., followed by breakfast preparation, gathering provisions, and a Jeep ride to our hunting location. We were going to hunt together since this was her first time trying to harvest a deer. I wanted to be there to help her, if she needed it, and to see the joy on her face when she harvested that first buck. It didn't take long.

A nice-sized buck that met our restrictions in size came into the area. Sally took her time, waited until the buck was standing broadside, took aim, and fired. The buck fell but jumped back up and ran into the trees. She was not worried because she knew she had made a good shot. We waited about 15 minutes, climbed down out of the stand, and went to where we felt like the buck had been standing. We found the trail, followed it for about 40 yards, and there was her first buck lying on its side, dead. We hugged, and she was so happy she almost exploded.

We hunted together, just like we bowled together, fished together, just like we did everything together. Our lives felt complete, and I could not be happier with her accomplishments. We were truly one together!

Looking back, it is tempting to believe that a life so full, so deeply shared, would somehow be protected from what lay ahead. We had weathered loss before, learned resilience, and built a marriage rooted in faith, trust, and togetherness. Nothing about our daily routines suggested that anything was wrong.

Yet trouble rarely arrives with a warning. It begins with the smallest disruptions—moments that seem harmless, easily explained, and quickly forgiven. At the time, we laughed them off. Only later would we understand that these were not isolated incidents, but the earliest whispers of a journey neither of us was prepared to take.

SIX

Subtle Signs of Trouble

Trouble doesn't give signs like rain,
so we must always be ready for it.
Ciannon Smart

Just before the time of COVID-19 in 2019, minor things began happening. None of these were setting off any genuine alarms with me, and Sally was always brushing them off. She would say, "I'm getting old." We would laugh, and I would tell her I did not think she was old in any way. She was my "Baby." She was the type who would never let our home get unorganized or dirty. She ensured it remained immaculate and orderly.

We lived in an area in Huntsville, Texas called Elkins Lake. It was primarily a golfing community with three 9-hole courses. We both enjoyed playing together. Elkins Lake was like our dream retirement area. We constantly remarked how we never thought we would live in as nice a place as this when we retired. We counted ourselves very blessed.

She was very organized, and so she always had every day of the week planned out completely.

Glimpse: Sally enjoyed having a consistent schedule both at home and in her social life.

On Sunday, we attended church together. Over the years, during one of my sporadic visits to church with Sally, I had rededicated my life to Christ, and my priorities had changed. From that point on, I became an avid student of the Word of God, changing the way I lived my life, and

58

always attending church on Sundays with her. We discussed my life and how it had changed for the better.

This led to conversations about the possibility of entering the ministry and becoming the pastor of a church. *Together* we made that decision, and I quickly went to work to become an ordained minister, which we *together* achieved.

Afterward, I had the pleasure of leading several small churches in the area. While I preached, Sally sang in the choir. On Sunday afternoons, we went home after church and lunch, loaded up in our golf cart, and played golf together.

Monday, I volunteered at the golf courses and sanded divots on hole number six for the Ravines course. She did laundry that morning, and upon my return from sanding, I helped her make the bed with the clean sheets.

Tuesday was ladies' golf day, so she played in the "Niners" competition. Sally headed this group, and she set up the type of competition they would play each Tuesday. On Tuesday mornings, I was in the Men's Bible Study. As the women were using the course, it was an ideal day for the study because the men couldn't tee off until approximately 11:00 a.m. We held our study at 8:00 a.m. and finished by 9:30 a.m. If any of the men wanted to play, it worked out time-wise. After the Bible study, I normally took the rest of the morning and worked on my golf game.

After she finished playing, Sally would usually inform me she was leaving, prompting me to collect my clubs and personal items before returning home to meet her. Sometimes we fixed lunch, normally a sandwich and chips, or we went out for lunch.

Our favorite place to go for lunch was Mayflower Bakery. They served a delicious chicken salad sandwich combo. It included a sandwich on your choice of bread, chips of your choice, a cookie of your choice, a pickle, and a medium drink of your choice. You could get all of this for $6.50 apiece—a price that couldn't be beat!

On Wednesdays, the men had the golf courses for a competition, which I usually competed in. That was also housecleaning day. Sally vacuumed and dusted the house, but would leave the ceiling fans for me to dust upon my return home from golf. Before leaving to play, I brought the vacuum up out of the garage and set it between the kitchen and the formal dining room.

Thursday was a day when we normally went up to Leona, Texas, for lunch with people from the church. Sally would check to see if Mary was planning to be there. If so, we went. On those rare occasions when Mary would not be at lunch, we stayed home. Then, later that afternoon, we would try to play golf together.

Friday, she had her women's Bible study that started at 9:00 a.m. and usually ended just before noon. Friday afternoon was usually spent around the house, with me mowing the yard and her gardening or pulling weeds. On Friday afternoons, we went to our bank because they gave away ice cream bars. We rarely missed the ice cream treats. Friday evening was "Grilled Hamburger Night" with French fries or tater tots.

Saturday, one of us seemed to be in a golf tournament of some kind, either a women's tournament, a men's tournament, or sometimes a couple's tournament. Saturday evening, typically, I prepared the sermon for church, and she listened and gave me constructive criticism.

ONE DAY, SHE came to me because she was having trouble figuring out what to do and how to line up the ladies for Tuesday morning "Niners Golf." I told her she needed to see Ray, the head golf professional and golf shop head, and ask him to help her. The first time, we went down together to meet him. Ray was more than happy to help her.

Sally's infectious personality was so beloved that anyone who knew her would readily help her. At that time, there was no cause for me to think any more about this. But a few months later, she came to me again and told me she did not feel comfortable continuing to run the Niner program.

"You've been doing this for several years," I told her. "It's probably time for someone else to take on that responsibility." I did not realize there was a bigger issue causing this problem.

What was happening was that when she explained the game for that Tuesday that she and Ray had set up, some ladies asked her questions. She could not figure out how to answer them and would have to ask Ray. This caused a problem with some ladies, and it bothered her. That was why she did not feel like she could do this for the Niners anymore.

One Wednesday, I came home after playing in the men's competition and noticed the vacuum had not been moved or used. I could tell it had not been used because it had a clear canister, which had to be emptied after every use (usually by me). This canister had nothing in it. When I went into the living room, I found her in her recliner, watching reruns of *Gunsmoke.* I asked if she had cleaned the house, and she looked at me with a slight bit of confusion. She then said she thought she would wait until I got home and we could do it together.

No problem. I cleaned the ceiling fans and then ran the vacuum while Sally dusted. In less than an hour, we were finished. Something felt different, but it did not seem to be a big deal at the time.

That same fall, we had a time when our weather was warmer than normal. She had the controls on her Toyota Camry set to air conditioning because of the warm weather. Then, like normal here in Texas, the weather changed, and suddenly we woke up to an unusually cool day. It was a Tuesday, so I went to the men's Bible study and then normally would go play golf. But since it was so cool, I came home right after the Bible study and was there when she came home.

She came into the house and told me something was wrong with the heater in her Camry. It was blowing cold air out of the vents in the dashboard. So I went out and started the car, and sure enough, the air was coming out of the vents, and it was *cold*. A glance at the controls showed that they were set on air conditioning, at maximum cold. I set them to heat and turned the temperature up with warm air coming out of the floor vents.

Returning inside, I asked her about the setting. She said she had done that, but nothing happened, so she put them back where they were. She told me those controls always confused her. I felt something was wrong, but she was smiling and wanted to go to lunch, so we took her car, and off to lunch we went.

The disturbing thing was that this car was a 2016, and she had operated the controls with no problem for four years. Something was definitely wrong, but I dismissed it. We had a chicken salad sandwich combo at our favorite lunch place, and then we went to the grocery store and did our weekly shopping.

THE NEXT WEEK, we took a trip to visit family in Wichita, Kansas, leaving after church on Sunday. We drove first to Johnna's house, arriving about 7:30 p.m. Johnna had decided several years ago to move back to Kansas in order to be closer to extended family. She had also found better job opportunities in the area. It was much cooler in Wichita than it was in Huntsville, so we stayed in most of the time unless we went to visit extended family.

Johnna needed to take one of her horses to an equine water treadmill. The horse enters a tub enclosure filled with warm water, with a treadmill on the bottom. The horse walks on this treadmill, which gives it much-needed exercise; this is especially helpful for older horses. Sally rode with her. When they returned to the house, she told me all about this whirlpool treadmill for horses.

While visiting Johnna, our granddaughter, her husband, and three children, our great-grandchildren, came to her house for dinner. Sally talked to them and greeted each one of them with her big hugs. She spoke with Kylie, the granddaughter, and asked how she was doing. Then she spoke to Cooper, our grandson-in-law, asking him the same question. Then, her attention turned to the great-grandchildren.

She asked each of them the same question, with the follow-up question of how they were doing in school. The issue came about when she would finish with one great-grandchild and go to another. Strangely, she asked the same questions repeatedly, as if she did not remember having talked to that child. I picked up on this, but it was time to sit down and eat, so everything changed.

EARLY-STAGE ALZHEIMER'S (MILD)

Observations: At first, a person remains independent and can drive, but they may notice memory gaps, such as forgetting words or the location of objects. Family and close friends may notice the changes, while the patient may pass them off as nothing. A doctor can diagnose this stage with specific diagnostic tools.

Memory, language, and thinking are the three primary domains affected by the progressive nature of Alzheimer's. Memory problems are often the first sign. However, individuals in the early stages of Alzheimer's exhibit symptoms beyond mere forgetfulness. Common early-stage symptoms include:

-Having trouble recalling words and names.
-Displaying general apathy
-Difficulty performing tasks in social settings
-Meeting challenges in following instructions

[cont'd next page]

-Forgetting what was just read
-Asking the same questions repeatedly
-Losing/misplacing valuable objects
-Struggling to plan and organize

What You Can Do: Focus on aspects of life that are most meaningful to them. Put legal, financial, and end-of-life plans in place while they can still take part in the decision-making process.

SEVEN

The Signs Intensify

*None of us wants to be reminded that dementia is
random, relentless, and frighteningly common.*
Laurie Graham

About a month after our trip to Wichita, we left for the Phoenix area to spend Thanksgiving with our daughter, Tonya, her husband, Juan, and her children. We left on Sunday after church and drove to Fort Stockton, Texas, where we spent the night at a hotel. The next morning, we were up early for breakfast at the hotel, and then we were on the road continuing our trip to Juan and Tonya's house.

While we were driving through New Mexico, Sally spotted some antelope, which she had never seen before, and she pointed to this enormous field of "deer." Looking out, I spotted the antelope and explained to her that those were not deer, but antelope. She remarked that she didn't think she had ever seen an antelope before. I didn't believe she had ever encountered an antelope previously, but I urged her to continue observing, as more were likely to appear, and indeed they did, much to her delight!

We arrived at the place we were staying in the Mesa area, close to our daughter's house. With five people living in their house, Juan and Tonya and their three children, they did not have an extra bedroom for us. Therefore, we rented a place nearby for the week. We called and told Tonya we were there and would be over as soon as we unloaded our stuff into the small rental house.

About 4:00 p.m., we pulled into their driveway. It would not be long until dinner, which would be at about 6:00 p.m. Maggie was there, and she hugged and kissed her grandmother, which caused Sally to just gleam with joy. Jack, their son, our grandson, was working and would not be home until after 9:00 p.m., so we would not see him until the next day. Emily, the oldest granddaughter, was also working and would not get home until about the same time, so we would see her the next day as well.

Maggie stuck to Sally, and no matter what she wanted, Maggie was on the job and took extremely good care of her grandmother. Sally enjoyed all of this attention. We ate dinner together, and then left and headed for the rental house because it had been a long day, and we were both tired.

The next morning, we found a little breakfast diner. We pulled up in front of this little egg place, parked the Camry, and went inside. The young lady who greeted us remarked on our being from Texas. She had spotted the license plate on the front of the car. We had an appetizing breakfast, and then we headed for Juan and Tonya's house.

All three of the grandchildren were there when we arrived, and we exchanged hugs with all of them. Maggie once again became glued to her grandmother, taking care of every need or want she might have. Sally talked to Jack and asked her normal questions. "Are you doing all right? How are you doing in school?" She asked the same questions of Emily. She and Maggie continued to be connected at the hip, and Maggie would not leave her alone.

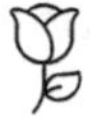 **Glimpse:** Sally had a way of connecting with others and making them feel special.

We ate lunch as a group, and then Jack and Emily had to head off to work. The next day was Thanksgiving Day, so everyone would be there, since both places where Jack and Emily worked would be closed for the day.

Juan had a new smoker, so he was trying his hand at smoking a turkey and a ham. Juan loved technology, so he connected his phone to the smoker via Bluetooth. He could control the temperature and the amount of smoke from his phone.

The cooking started right after we arrived that morning. I found Juan's explanation of controlling the smoker via his phone to be quite interesting. We were scheduled to eat at about 4:00 p.m., so things were going well. He had temperature probes in the turkey, as well as the ham, monitoring the internal temperatures of both items simultaneously. His phone would tell him, by beeping, when the desired temperature was reached.

Maggie and Sally were together, and Maggie had her grandmother engaged in some sort of game on the iPad. She kept herself entertained and made Sally very happy with all the attention she was getting from her granddaughter.

The meal was ready on time, and we all sat down together, all seven of us. Juan blessed the meal, and we devoured the grand feast before us. Naturally, we all ate more than we needed, even Sally, so after the meal, everyone was full and quiet. Jack disappeared into his bedroom and took a nap, something I think several of us thought about. Still, Jack was the only one to take advantage of the situation.

We left around 7:30 p.m. and headed for our place. We were both very full, so we were asleep by 9:30 p.m. The next morning, I woke up at about 6:30 a.m. Sally was still sleeping soundly, so I went to shave and take my shower. After doing so and drying off, I heard Sally screaming, "John, where are you?"

I hurried into the bedroom from the bathroom and asked her what was wrong. She was crying and did not know where she was, and she thought I had left her alone! I calmed her down, hugged her, and told her I would not leave her. After giving her a reassuring kiss, she finally calmed down. At that moment, I knew something was wrong with my Baby!

THE REST OF the trip was uneventful, and we left the following Tuesday for the two-day drive home to Huntsville. We drove for a little over two hours, and we pulled into a Love's fuel stop to fill up the car with gasoline and use the restrooms. She told me she was going inside to use the bathroom.

"Wait for me inside," I said, and she agreed. Then I filled the car with gasoline, paid at the pump, and went inside to use the restroom and meet Sally.

Upon arriving at the entrance to the restrooms, she was not standing there, so I went on into the men's restroom. After finishing and exiting the restroom, she was still not waiting at the entrance. In a couple of minutes, a lady came towards the restroom. I approached her and asked if she would look for Sally in the women's restroom, and she agreed. She went inside and checked for Sally, but soon came out and said that she was not there. A panic I had never experienced came over me. At that instant, a Loves' employee came up and asked if I was John.

"Yes, I am." He told me he thought that my wife was at the cashier, and she seemed lost.

I thanked him and rushed to the cashier area, and there she was with her hands folded and scared. I put my arms around her and asked her if she wanted a fancy cup of coffee. She responded, "That would be nice."

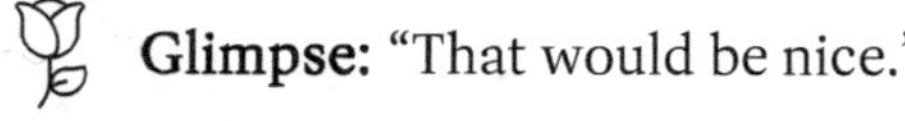 **Glimpse:** "That would be nice."

We paid for the coffees, then headed to the car and continued our trip home. From that time on, when we stopped for gasoline, she stayed beside me while I filled the car with gasoline. Then we would go to the restroom areas together.

On the rest of the trip home, I noticed that when a car would pass us on her side when we were in a town, she would get very nervous. It was as if the car passing her scared her or caught her off guard. We made it home to Huntsville on Wednesday afternoon, went to the store together, washed the car, went to the mailbox, and then went home for the night.

THE NEXT TUESDAY, we both returned home after playing golf, and she asked if I would assist her with her short game and putting practice. We loaded the golf cart back up and headed for the practice green down by the clubhouse. When we got there, I explained we were going to putt first, and I was heading over to set things up for her to practice. She told me, "That would be nice," and I headed for the green.

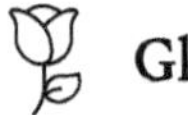 **Glimpse:** "That would be nice."

No one was there using the green, so I picked out a hole in the center and set up the circle putting drill from three feet. From the hole, you measure out about three feet, and you make a circle around the hole. Then, you pick out five spots around that circle and place five golf balls on them. The idea of the drill was that she now had five putts, all from three feet, but from different directions to the hole. This technique worked in helping the golfer concentrate on making, or trying to make, all five putts.

When she came down to where the drill was set up, she was carrying her six iron and not her putter.

"Why did you bring the six-iron instead of your putter?" I asked.

She responded by saying she thought that was what I said to bring. I told her it was OK and took her six-iron back to her golf bag and exchanged it for her putter. We spent some time putting in, and she did

OK, but nothing compared to what she usually does. She told me she was tired and wanted to just go home.

THE FOLLOWING SATURDAY, after playing with my regular group of men, we had a birthday celebration for one of them. Sally and the other wives came to the clubhouse restaurant for lunch, the gift giving, and of course, birthday cake. One of the guys' wives, Barbara, came to me after we finished and asked if I knew that Sally was having a tough time playing on Tuesdays.

"What do you mean?" I asked.

She told me Sally did not know which club to use. She would often carry an iron up to the tee box instead of her driver. While most ladies offered support, some were annoyed by Sally's confusion and expressed their displeasure, which in turn upset her. I explained that I was aware of something going on. But I lacked clarity on exactly what was happening.

EIGHT

Getting a Diagnosis

---

*The tragedy of dementia is that it robs us of the
ability to hold onto our dearest memories, but the
person we love is still there, beneath it all.*
MERYL COMER

That afternoon, I went online to our medical group and made an appointment for her on Monday morning with her primary care doctor. Via the appointment form, I explained my concerns about Sally's mental acuity. Then I tried to prepare Sally for her appointment.

"Sally, you have a doctor's appointment on Monday with your regular doctor."

"Why?"

"It's just a routine check-up."

"I'm fine. I don't need an appointment."

"O.K. Well, it's just a check-up. We should probably go anyway."

At the appointment on Monday morning, the doctor, whom she had been seeing for about two years, recognized something was wrong almost immediately. She gave Sally a simple cognitive test, and out of the 10 questions, she only answered one correctly. She referred Sally to a neurologist, Dr. Sachs, and we set up an appointment with him for the following week.

Sally was not happy about that, but when we arrived home, I talked to her about what was going on. She admitted that she was having a problem, but that she was all right.

"We're going to find out what the problem is," I told her. "Then we'll figure out what to do together." She relaxed, smiled, and asked me to hold her.

The next week, we went to see Dr. Sachs, and I explained what I had seen and what had been reported to me. He performed a basic cognitive test with her, and out of the 30 questions and drawings that were part of the test, she did not answer any of them correctly.

He told me that, in his medical opinion, she should not be driving, and he asked if I had a medical power of attorney or a durable power of attorney for her. I told him I had both, and she had both for me. He told me he was going to schedule three different brain scans at Saint Luke's Hospital. When he had the results, his nurse would inform us and get us immediately back in for the consultation.

THE TESTS TOOK place the next week, all three in one day, at Saint Luke's Hospital. Dr. Sachs' nurse called us in about three days to schedule us back in to see him and review the results. We went to see him on a Tuesday at 11:00 a.m., at the Kelsey-Seybold Clinic, where we had seen him before.

We went into the room, and in no time, Dr. Sachs came in and sat down. He asked Sally what her name was. She told him, "Sally." Then he asked her what her last name was. She looked at me because she did not know. He told her it was OK. He moved me over where I could see his computer screen, and he started going through the test results.

We looked at the first scan, and he told me she had not had a stroke nor did she have bleeding on her brain, all good things. Then he showed another picture of her skull and the position of her brain. He pointed out to me that there was a small space between the skull and her brain. The abnormality signaled that her brain was decreasing in size.

Then, the third scan was like an MRI of the brain, where we looked at slices of the brain. In the frontal lobe, there were two dark spots on both sides. He explained this was Alzheimer's. The brain shrinking was caused by dementia, which is the overall disease. He told me she was most likely in late-stage two or early-stage three of the disease. He was very kind, and he explained that there was no cure for this, and it would eventually take her life.

He asked me if I had received his letter stating she was in cognitive decline. I said "Yes." He told me he would make notes on her chart, which I could retrieve, concerning everything we had discussed. In his opinion, he thought she had dementia/Alzheimer's. He told me to activate the medical/financial power of attorney and attach this letter to it, making it official. Before we left, he gave me a list of books and online resources where one could learn about this disease.

Obtaining The Initial Diagnosis

What to Expect: Receiving an Alzheimer's diagnosis is the culmination of a roller coaster of emotions. Acknowledging and understanding these feelings can aid in the coping process. Many patients will experience anger, relief, denial, numbness, fear, and a sense of loss. Obtaining a diagnosis allows the patient and their family to move forward emotionally and practically as everyone prepares. There is no "correct" approach for dealing with an Alzheimer's diagnosis. Some may need personal time to mourn, while others may benefit from staying engaged in their favorite activities.

What You Can Do: If questions arise after receiving the diagnosis, there are several reliable online resources. Again, you're not alone, and it is worth it to find support!

ON THE WAY home from Dr. Sachs' visit, she was in total silence and was looking down at her hands. The trip home took about 30 minutes, and for 25 minutes she did not say a word. I could tell she was shaken up about this visit to Dr. Sachs. She may have been trying to make some sort of sense out of all that was happening to her, but couldn't.

We were just about home, and she finally said, "John, when we get home, I want you to do me a favor."

"Honey, if I can, I will do it for you."

"Since I am not worth anything anymore, I want you to load one of your guns and shoot me in the head."

I can't describe what I felt at that moment. My desire to hold her and declare my love was overshadowed by the task of driving.

ALZHEIMER'S/DEMENTIA RESOURCES

-www.alz.org
-www.alzheimers.gov
-www.nia.nih.gov
-www.mayoclinic.org

IMPORTANT DATES IN THE ALZHEIMER'S COMMUNITY:

-**June** is Alzheimer's & Brain Awareness Month (represented by the color purple and the Forget-Me-Not flower)
-**September 21** is World Alzheimer's Day
-**September** is World Alzheimer's Month
-**November** is recognized by some organizations as Alzheimer's Awareness Month (represented by the color teal)

In-Home Support

Early in January, we had dentist appointments to get our teeth cleaned and checked. I had made the appointments, telling the lady on the phone about my wife's situation, and asked if we could be seen at the same time. She assured me it could happen, so we went to the dentist for our appointments.

The dentist's office was in a mall in Conroe, Texas, about 20 minutes from our home. I parked close to the door because we were some of the very first appointments for that day. We checked in at the desk, and we went and sat down in the waiting area. Soon, Sally was summoned, and then my name was called right after. We both received a clean bill of dental health.

But Sally, who finished her appointment first, was not in the waiting room, so I went to the front desk. Upon asking if she was still with the dentist, they referred me to the waiting area. There were several patients there, and a couple of them had small children, so they had probably made Sally nervous. The people in the waiting area saw Sally for a few minutes, but she told one of them she was going out to our truck to wait. However, she did not have a key to unlock the truck, and when I looked, she was not near it.

I told the manager of the dentist's office about my problem. It was a little upsetting because they knew Sally had dementia/Alzheimer's. The manager offered to help look for her, so we split off in two different directions, combing the mall.

A slight panic came over me. Just as I was getting ready to call 911, a voice hollered my name. It was the manager. She had found Sally sitting on the curb crying because she was lost and did not know how to get back to the dentist's office. I gave her a big hug and told her everything was all right.

She looked at me with a look in her eyes that told me she was in a state of total fear. We went and got into the truck and headed home.

"Did you just decide to go shopping?" I asked.

"I guess that's what happened."

That day, I put a tracker on her phone, ensuring her phone was in her purse or pocket anytime we went anywhere.

AFTER THIS INCIDENT, I called Dr. Sachs' office. He ordered a prescription for Sally that would help with anxiety and episodes of continual crying. Wanting to know everything about this disease, I scoured Dr. Sachs' recommended websites and books. I needed help because trying to be with her and take care of her 24 hours a day was difficult at best. The last thing she needed was for me to collapse or do something wrong.

Dr. Sachs' nurse recommended a few agencies, including Pam's Senior Helpers. To learn more about their programs and their ability to help Sally and me, I arranged meetings with each of them.

Of the three recommendations given by Dr. Sachs, Pam's made the best impression. Plus, their service was recommended by our neurologist's nurse. We set up daily hours, starting with five days a week, five hours a day. A friend had called me and offered to arrange for several friends from the Bible study to be with Sally on Saturdays. It seemed a plan was falling into place.

CARE FOR THE CARETAKER

Caregiving can be fulfilling and meaningful work, but it is not without its challenges. Caring for yourself is important for maintaining your own physical and emotional well-being. Ensuring you have a support system around you is a great place to start. Other ways to practice self-care as a caregiver include:

-Joining a support group
-Taking short, daily breaks
-Exercising in ways you enjoy
-Spending time with loved ones
-Processing your emotions honestly
-Setting time aside for hobbies

Caretakers often worry about the future, in case something impedes their ability to provide care. One way to relieve this anxiety is to prepare for the unknown. Put together a backup plan by collecting and organizing information about your patient—emergency phone numbers, behavioral challenges, favorite activities, routines, local organizations, and nearby long-term care facilities. Being prepared for the unknown will ease stress and keep you present.

Sally was excited about the proposal. Pam brought Gloria by to meet her on a Saturday. Sally liked her a lot, so I felt comfortable with the situation and felt like it would work.

Gloria arrived on Monday morning, bright and early at 7:00 a.m. Sally instantly recognized her with a hug, and the bond was sealed. The plan was set. Gloria would stay with Sally until noon. Her routine would be the same every weekday. This schedule gave me time to run errands, teach the men's Bible study, and even allowed for a little golf if I was home by noon.

We worked together to take care of her, and Gloria appreciated that. She also noticed the little things that Sally needed. For instance, her legs were dry and needed some moisturizing lotion. Sally had plenty of it in several brands. Gloria took her into the bedroom, took off her pants, and went to work rubbing the lotion on her legs. Sally's love languages were quality time and acts of service. Her face would light up when Gloria was massaging her legs.

When I left to run errands, Gloria had everything under control. When Sally went into one of her episodes of crying, Gloria embraced her and talked to her, which was what I had learned worked best for those times. Gloria had a lot of knowledge about this disease because she had cared for others like Sally for years. Gloria always knew how to help me when I had issues involving her.

Gloria was with us for about six months. During that time, she only missed three days at the most. Usually, that was for a doctor's appointment or a dentist's appointment, but those times over the six months were very rare. Gloria kept me updated on things while on my errands.

The disease was progressing, and I knew that it was getting close to the time when she would have to be placed in a skilled nursing facility, which wasn't my first choice. With the help of Gloria, we were able to care for her for at least two months past the time she should have probably been at a facility.

Gloria told me that after I left, she would be fine for an hour or so, but then she started looking for me. She walked around the house, going from room to room, sometimes calling out my name. She would ask Gloria, "Is John coming back?"

Gloria always responded, "Has there ever been a time when he did not come to you?" That would put her at ease and would make the rest of the time easier until I returned home. She started watching the reruns of *Gunsmoke*, with Matt Dillon as the marshal of Dodge City, Kansas. She would watch that show for hours on end, and it helped pass the time.

Upon arriving home, we would say goodbye to Gloria. Before she left, she'd always say goodbye to Sally, whom she referred to as "Momma," by saying, "I will see you in the morning, Momma."

At times, Sally would say, "I'll be looking for you."

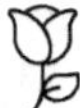 **Glimpse**: Sally often responded to others with "I'll be looking for you."

MIDDLE-STAGE ALZHEIMER'S (MODERATE)

Observations: This is typically the longest stage, sometimes lasting years. Dementia symptoms become more pronounced. The patient may act in unexpected ways or become easily frustrated and angry. They may have more difficulty expressing thoughts and need more assistance performing routine tasks. Middle-stage symptoms include:

-forgetting events or personal history (e.g., address, phone #, etc.)
-experiencing confusion regarding times and locations
-wandering to the point of becoming lost
-being moody or withdrawn in social settings
-requiring help to choose proper clothing
-struggling to control bladder and bowels
-exhibiting sleep pattern changes

[cont'd next page]

Other personality and behavioral changes may also appear, such as suspicion, delusion, and compulsive behaviors.

What You Can Do: The patient may still participate in some daily activities with assistance. Find out what they enjoy doing and simplify the task. Respite care allows caregivers to take a welcome break.

TEN

The Move to a Skilled Nursing Facility

> *Though those with Alzheimer's might forget us, we*
> *as a society must remember them.*
> SCOTT KIRSCHENBAUM, FILMMAKER

As Sally continued to progress with the disease, Gloria told me we were nearing the time to look for a skilled nursing facility. Neither one of us wanted to see that happen. In order to help, my sister Martha came into town, and she stayed with us, which Sally enjoyed.

Four skilled nursing homes in the area had openings and would accept a Medicaid-pending resident. Martha and I went to visit these places, not really knowing what to look for or what questions to ask. We looked to make sure it seemed the facility had enough staff, but we really did not understand how they operated, so everything seemed fine to us.

We both settled on a facility that was the largest and it also happened to be the newest. The only drawback we could see was that it was 30 to 45 minutes from our home. *That's not a problem*, I thought, not knowing how much time the drive would take. But the decision was made. The letter from Dr. Sachs was sent to the facility with his recommendation that she be placed there, and that she had been diagnosed with dementia/Alzheimer's.

The date was set. Gloria and Pam were informed of our decision to place her in a skilled nursing facility. Johnna came down the week before the day when we were to take her to her new place of residence. Neither one of us was looking forward to that day. Although I was unsure of how Sally would manage the situation, the thought of abandoning her there would present a challenge for me. I was thankful for Johnna's presence and support.

WHEN THE DAY came for her move, we loaded up the car. She was looking forward to the drive because it was an adventure for her. We arrived, and Vicky, the director of nursing, took Johnna and her mother back to her room. She started normal checking of her blood pressure, heart rate, and listening to her heart and lungs—all was well. Having finished the paperwork and paid, I went to the room, feeling pleased that Sally and her roommate were the same age and that her roommate also had dementia.

Sally was thinking something was different, and when I came into her room, she looked at me and said, "Don't leave me."

"You know that I will always come back to be with you."

Her roommate took hold of her hand and suggested they go to the activities room for an afternoon of music and singing. Sally loved music and singing. She looked at us and told us she would see us later, and they left and headed for the activities center.

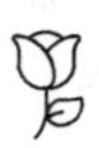 **Glimpse:** She always had a way of finding and making friends, and everyone who met her loved her. That's how I knew she would be all right.

Johnna and I looked at each other and decided it was time for us to go. We felt like she was in good hands and well taken care of, as well as being involved in the multitude of various activities that went on almost non-stop every day.

When we got into the truck to head home, Johnna asked, "How are you feeling?"

"Not very well." I started to cry. It wasn't a decision that had come easily.

Johnna placed her hand on my arm. "Same with me." After a minute or two, we decided to stop off at a place we had spotted on the way to the facility and grab dinner.

We visited Sally the next day, and when we arrived, she was out by the nurses' station talking to one of the nurses. We walked almost right up to her before she saw us. When she saw us, she put her hands out and called me "Dads," and we hugged, and I kissed her. She then turned to Johnna and gave her a big hug. She told us she knew we were coming to see her.

I told her, "You know I always come to you."

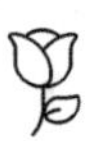 **Glimpse:** Her eyes sparkled, and she told us she knew we would come to her. This sparkle in her eyes would provide a special peek into her heart in the weeks and months to come.

From my observations, she was all right, but she was also trying to adjust to her new surroundings. The nurse at the nurses' station told us she had been helping her with some papers.

"Have you found a new job?" I asked her.

Sally smiled really big. "They needed help, so I was just helping."

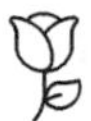 **Glimpse:** That was the way she was throughout her entire life— always trying to help others.

We went to the lounge area and sat down at a table. "What have you been doing?"

She couldn't remember, but when we brought up the activities, she said, "Oh, I really enjoy those!"

"Tell us about the times when they play the music, and you get to sing along."

Her eyes sparkled, and a big smile came across her face. "Oh, I know almost all the songs. I clap and sing out loud with the other peoples." She called the residents in her group "peoples" because she could not remember their names.

Sally finally started talking about the various things she could do. She really liked the "lady," which was the name she gave to the nurse in physical therapy. She told us she was really sweet.

It seemed like we had not been with her for very long, when actually we had been there for over three hours. Her roommate came over and told her it was time to play bingo. She looked at us and told us she would see us later. We hugged and kissed her, and I told her to watch for us because we would come back to be with her. She smiled and just said, "I know you will come to me."

Glimpse: She often smiled and responded, "I know you will come to me."

Johnna and I left, and when we got into the truck to head home, she looked at me and told me she thought her mother was doing fine. I agreed. It seemed that the more we were losing Sally physically and mentally, the more glimpses of her we would see. That allowed us to feel good about the situation, or as good as we could.

As Sally's condition worsened, the poem below became more significant to me.

My eyes do see, my ears do hear,
I am still me, so let's be clear.
My memory may fade, my walk may slow,
But I am "me" inside, don't let me go.

Our visit on Sunday went well. It seemed like Sally was really getting into all the activities they had for the residents. She told us when we arrived after church that their service was different from our church. She liked it fine because they sang lots of songs. She loved to sing songs, especially the hymns of the church.

However, on Monday morning, Vicky called to let me know they were going to place an ankle monitor on Sally after she had taken off several times to wander the halls. She had not tried to leave, but they did not want that to happen. The ankle monitor would cause an alarm to sound if she tried to open a door and leave the building. I was told that probably half of the residents had them and that it was fairly normal.

How Do Memory Care Nurses Minimize Risks For Their Patients?

Because of the unique challenges for people with cognitive impairments, certain risks are amplified in memory-care settings. These include elopement, dehydration, falls, and other concerns. When properly trained, facility staff use approaches to mitigate patient dangers. Family members not accustomed to these strategies may find them alarming. Here are important protocols used in well-trained facilities:

-Keeping the environment safe, including securing the entrances with a check-in desk and placing alarms on windows and doors if a patient attempts to wander off unsupervised.
-Monitoring and surveillance systems are frequently employed by facilities to track a client's location.
-Observing changes in the patient's eating habits. All staff members, including cafeteria workers and aides, must note any changes in the patient's ability to swallow or chew, as these pose a potential risk of choking and aspiration. Immediate adjustments can be made to puree or chop the food and minimize risk.

Later on, that same day, Vicky called again, and she told me she was going to schedule a meeting with a psychiatrist to evaluate her medications. She was only taking one drug, which helped her with her anxiety. Agreeing to the visit, I was still a little concerned, being warned about psychiatrists and their wanting to prescribe a pill for everything. A friend of mine, a retired MD, told me to be wary of psychiatrists. He told me they had "a pill to fix everything."

The next Monday morning at about 9:00 a.m., I met with the director of the facility, LaTisha, as well as Vicky, the psychiatrist, Sally, and me. The doctor began by describing the drug that she was currently taking.

"Mr. Burchell, are you aware of the potential side effects of the drug your wife is taking? On rare occasions, it has expedited the death of some who have dementia/Alzheimer's."

"Yes, it has been explained, but the benefits we experience seem to outweigh the risks."

"Well, we have a new medication that will do the same thing without those potential side effects. Would you like to try it?"

"Yes, let's do that."

"There is also a medication that will help with 'Sundown Syndrome.'"

"O.K. Let's see if that will help her then."

She would go to bed at night and go to sleep, but in just an hour or so, she would wake up, get out of bed, and wander throughout the facility. Therefore, they had placed an ankle monitor on her to alert the nurses and aides if she tried to leave the facility.

So far, she had never tried to leave. Mainly, she would just go to the nurses' station and talk to them. I did not see a problem with that, but that is not something the staff wanted to have to do. She would eventually go back to bed, but she could be up and awake as much as four or five hours. The doctor explained that she needed to sleep, and this would calm her so she would stay asleep at night.

The two new medications were started that very day. We spent the rest of the morning looking at pictures in some children's books that she liked. At about 11:30 a.m., an aide came and told us it was time for lunch in the dining room. We went to the table where her regular group ate. Immediately after the meal, they would clean up the dining hall and move to the activities room to sing songs and listen to music.

"It looks like you are going to be busy the rest of the day!" She agreed, so I kissed her goodbye and told her I would be back to see her.

Glimpse: She gave me the look of happiness, smiled really big, and told me she would watch for me to come to her.

My normal routine was to visit every other day, like Monday, Wednesday, Friday, and Sunday after church service. Time to her meant nothing anymore. To her, it was all about what activity they were getting ready for, meals, bathing, naptime, or bedtime. That was her day, and she seemed to do well at this facility.

ON MY NEXT visit, they were just finishing up their music. We spotted each other at the same time. Again, Sally responded with her huge smile and greeting.

Glimpse: She gave me a huge smile and stuck her hands out to greet me with a hug. She told me she knew I would come to her.

Sally seemed to be having a little bit of an issue with her attention span. It was very short.

"Would you like to lie down and rest?" She indicated that it sounded like a pleasant idea.

We went to her room, and I helped put her into bed. After covering her up and kissing her, she went right to sleep. After about an hour of sitting by her bedside, I got up to leave.

On my way out of the facility, I saw Vicky. "Sally seems to have changed. Can you tell me what's going on?"

"She's just adjusting to the new medications. Otherwise, everything is fine."

On my way home, thoughts swirled in my head about my Sally. We had been together for almost fifty years as husband and wife, and my mind was going down memory lane. For all those years, we had never really been apart except for the times I went to school to get my degree in theology. And there were a few hunting trips where we did not go together, as well as a ladies' bowling tournament that traveled all over the state of Texas.

How she loved to be in the boat fishing, but we did not have to fish. Some of the greatest times on the boat were the evenings when we lived in Crystal Beach on the canal. We would get into the boat, grab some drinks and snacks, and head for a place in East Galveston Bay. We just sat in the boat, faced west, and watched the sunset together.

It always amazed both of us when we watched the sunset how each was different and how each one was so special to us. Those quiet moments together in the boat, in a deer stand, walking the beach, or just anywhere we happened to be, were unforgettable. All we needed was each other and the presence of our Lord. We were filled with joy!

UPON RETURNING TO see her the next Saturday, our neighbors, Tommy and Connie, called to ask if they could stop in on their way to Lake Charles in about an hour. They were welcome to come, and Sally would be so excited to see them.

As I walked around looking for her, she was in the main room, listening to gospel hymns. I gave her a big hug and immediately noticed she was in a wheelchair. After a few minutes, we left that group and headed for the front visitation area to meet our friends. On the way, I questioned her about the wheelchair. "Tell me about the wheelchair. Do you feel like you need it?"

"I've been having some balance issues, so it's better to spend time in it." When she was talking, she appeared to be slurring her words a little. It was not bad, but it was evident that she was having some problems. With this disease, things constantly seemed to change from day to day, and I was learning to accept this.

We sat together on a big, overstuffed loveseat. When Tommy and Connie arrived in the visitation lounge, Sally immediately spotted them and beamed. She said, "Well, look who's here!" Then she perked right up and started talking to them.

"How do you like this new place?"

"It's OK, but I'd rather be home."

After about thirty minutes, she started to fade. Our friends told her they needed to get back on the road to Lake Charles, sharing hugs, and she told them she would be looking for them to come to see her again. Right after they left, she told me she wanted to rest for a bit, so I took her to her room.

When I helped her get into bed, she smiled at me and said, "I love you."

"I love you, too."

"I know you do." Right after that, she went to sleep. I stayed beside her for a little while longer and just looked at her. This disease was killing her, and there was nothing that could be done about that. My only wish was to experience our remaining time together fully.

🌷 **Glimpse:** She often responded to "I love you" with, "I know you do."

AFTER CHURCH THE next day, I headed for the nursing home to spend the afternoon with my baby. While I was driving and eating my packed lunch, she was having her lunch and then going to music.

Upon entering the music room, she was still in her wheelchair, but something was wrong. She was not sitting up straight but was slumped over to one side. As I helped her sit up straight, she looked at me, and something was not right.

"Are you all right?"

She just smiled and said, "I'll be all right, don't worry." When she talked, she was again slurring her words, which concerned me.

🌷 **Glimpse:** Sally often reassured others with the words, "I'll be all right."

The rest of the visit was spent on the loveseat with her head on my shoulder. With my arm around her, I told her about church. Sally was sleeping, but it didn't matter as we were together. When the aide came to get her at about 5:00 p.m. for dinner, she awoke and seemed to be better. She must have just been tired. We hugged and kissed, then I told her I loved her, and she was taken to the dining hall.

THE IMAGE OF my Sally in the wheelchair, slumped over, didn't sit right with me. Gloria would know. When I called her, she told me she had Tuesday off and would be glad to spend the day with Sally and give me a report of what she thought.

She went on Tuesday as planned and spent most of the day with Sally. Vicky called and asked if I knew Gloria was there with Sally.

"Yes, I asked her to visit Sally and report back with her observations. If she observed anything concerning, especially with her medication, I wanted to know."

Vicky was not very pleased. She acted like I was trying to prove something was going on that was improper. "Are you unhappy with her care? Do you think something is going on that is improper?"

"That is not my intent, but if that were to happen, I would want a trained professional nurse on my side." That ended my conversation with Vicky.

That evening, Gloria reached out concerning what she witnessed during the day she spent with Sally. She still remembered her from the time she was her primary caregiver. She said Sally was still her sweet self, but was being over-medicated, in her professional opinion. She explained that some nursing homes do that to residents who will not stay in their rooms, especially at night. Overmedicating the resident can cause them to sleep all night, even though it is not a natural sleep, but they will not get up and wander the halls.

The wandering, to most nurses at this type of facility, is not really a problem. Normally, the residents do not try to leave and normally do not cause any actual problems. Sally was one who just wanted something to do or someone to talk to.

But occasionally, a nurse may take classes online at night, and that nurse may not want any interference with their online classes. If that is the case, depending on how the doctor writes the order for the sleep aid, that nurse will administer extra doses of the medication, causing the resident to comply with their orders to go to bed and go to sleep.

According to what Gloria found, by looking at the orders, the doctor had written the order with the phrase, "every eight hours *or as needed*." It is the "or as needed" that becomes the issue. Since the drug prescribed for sleep did not keep Sally asleep, the "as needed" came into play. This is when a larger dose of the drug is administered. In Sally's condition, her bodily ability to metabolize the drug was very slow, and consequently, the next day, she would be groggy and incoherent.

"Thank you, Gloria, for *all* the information."

"You are welcome. You might want to consider moving Sally to another nursing facility." She gave me the name of one near my home. She knew the director of that nursing facility and assured me that this practice of overmedicating residents did not happen there because the director would not allow it to happen.

ELEVEN

Crisis at the Facility

*The true measure of a man is how he treats someone
who can do him absolutely no good.*
SAMUEL JOHNSON

The next morning, I called Focused Care and inquired if they had a bed available for a Medicaid-pending resident, which they did. My plan that day was to begin working on getting my wife transferred to their facility—first, a meeting with Vicky at the current facility needed to take place. I also asked that LaTisha, along with their staff social worker, be present. It was arranged for later that day.

Upon arrival, Vicky greeted me. The meeting would take place in their meeting room, so we headed that way. She was asking numerous questions, which I explained would be answered in the presence of LaTisha and the facility's social worker. The meeting started just a few minutes late because LaTisha was on a phone call. She finally came into the room, but it seemed like a long wait. In actuality, it was only about 15 minutes.

I started by telling them what Gloria had found and what she had reported to me. LaTisha expressed that it was not a problem for residents who wandered to be treated with kindness and respect. My concerns were brought up about the medication lists and how, on this one nurse's shift, she was always given extra medication because of the "as needed" part of the order. LaTisha asked Vicky if she was aware of this? She was not and said she would address it with Helen, the nurse in question.

I let them know my plan to relocate my wife to another facility. The social worker said that would not be a problem. She wanted to know where the facility was and the name of the facility, then she said she would go to her office and start that process immediately. LaTisha tried to stop her, but the social worker told her it would be in the best interest of the facility to expedite this because of the information I had in my possession.

This really did not sit well with LaTisha. Evidently, these types of transfers do not look good for the facility and for her. I told Vicky to stop giving Sally the sleep medication immediately, but to continue the anxiety medication at the same level. She said that would happen just as soon as the meeting ended, and it did.

After the meeting ended, Sally was at the nurse's station. I asked her what she was doing, and she said she was helping them "do things." The papers she had, about 10 pieces of paper, were blank and had nothing on them, but it was fine for Sally because she was helping "organize them for the nurse." Sally and I spent the rest of that morning and afternoon walking and talking without her wheelchair.

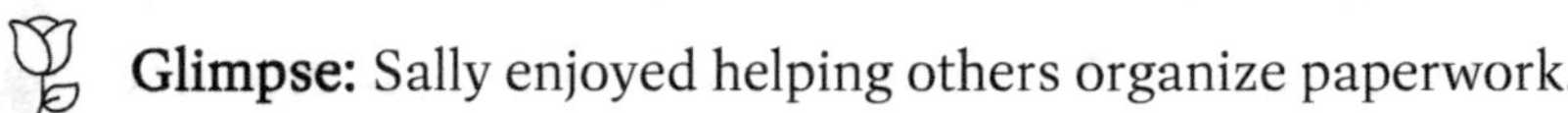 **Glimpse:** Sally enjoyed helping others organize paperwork.

It was obvious that Helen had not worked the night before, so Sally did not get extra medication. When it was time for the evening meal, the aide came to get Sally. She smiled at me and said, "Things are going to be all right!"

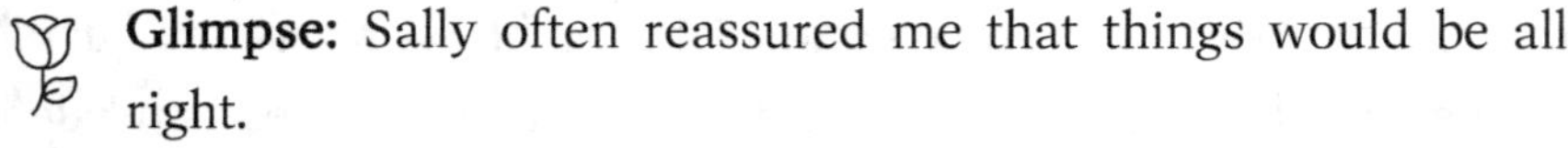 **Glimpse:** Sally often reassured me that things would be all right.

COMFORTABLE WITH THE outcome of the day, my trip home went by quickly. Arriving home around 8:00 p.m., I changed into comfy clothes and watched some *Monday Night Football* on television. At about 9:00 p.m., my phone rang. It was the nursing home.

As soon as I picked up the phone, someone started yelling at me. Sally was in the background, crying uncontrollably. The nurse, Helen, told me that if I did not talk to my wife and settle her down, she was going to use restraints on her to keep her in bed. Of course, I refused the demand for restraints. Sally was not a danger to anyone or herself. Yes, she might walk through the halls at night, but she would not do any harm to anyone or anything.

I asked Helen to hand the phone to Sally so I could speak with her. "It's your God-da##'d husband!" Helen yelled at Sally, telling her to speak on the phone.

When Sally picked up the phone, she was crying. "Sally, it's John. Nothing is going to happen to you."

She said she was afraid of that mean lady and that the lady was going to hurt her. I continued, "Is there anyone else in the room with you, Sally?" She told me the aide was there. "Give her the phone so that I can talk to her."

Upon answering, the aide, Lisa, stated she recalled helping Sally the day before, shortly before leaving for the night. Lisa informed me she would take care of Sally and station herself outside Sally's room. That way, if Sally woke up for any reason, Lisa would be there to take care of things. I thanked her and gave her my phone number, and asked her to call me if anything went wrong. If not, I would be there the following morning.

After tossing and turning all night, I showered and got dressed, then went into the kitchen. Making my coffee and breakfast, I read my Bible devotional, prayed, and felt ready for the day, not knowing what the situation would be when I arrived at the nursing home. That afternoon, our daughter, Johnna, was flying in and needed me to get her from the airport, which was close to the facility.

When I arrived at the nursing home that morning, Lisa was still on duty. Thanking her for her help, she told me that Helen had come to Sally's room very early to test her for COVID-19. Lisa said that Sally had tested positive and was now in quarantine. I went into the room anyway to see my Baby.

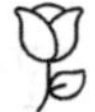 **Glimpse:** Sally smiled and told me she knew I would come to her.

While hugging and telling her I loved her and would always be there, she seemed fine. But she told me the mean lady had come in and hurt her nose. I told her to stay in the room and that I would be back in a few minutes.

Vicky was not present in the facility as she had apparently contracted COVID-19 herself. I went to LaTisha's office and informed her about my experience with being cursed at by Helen. As a pastor, I really did not appreciate people using God's name in vain, especially when they used it to curse me. I demanded a meeting with Helen. LaTisha informed me she would handle the situation with Helen. My response was that I intended to call the Houston Police and file charges against Helen.

LaTisha immediately asked me to give her a chance to deal with this before I filed charges. Agreeing to wait, I returned to my wife's room and helped her eat her breakfast. She did not seem to be sick, and she was not displaying any symptoms of COVID-19. No sore throat, no elevated body temperature, no coughing, no runny nose, no symptoms whatsoever.

About that time, right after we finished Sally's breakfast, LaTisha came into the room. She had on a gown and was wearing a mask. She told me she had the police on the phone, and the officer wanted to talk to me. When I took the phone, the officer introduced himself as Officer Raymond. He asked me to describe what had happened. I passed along what was discussed on the call regarding my wife and Helen's verbal abuse toward me. LaTisha told me to keep talking and excused herself, telling me she would be right back. The officer asked if I was alone in the room. At that point, we were.

He indicated they would arrive shortly, but he informed me that this wasn't the first complaint of its kind they'd received about the nurse and the facility. He also asked if my wife had been tested for COVID-19. Although Helen had said it was positive, my wife didn't appear to be sick.

He told me he recommended that I go and get two test kits and test for it myself. He told me Sally would probably test negative. This facility had a reputation for testing certain residents for COVID-19, claiming they were positive, but having no symptoms occurring after the test. Five days later, they would test negative. I asked Sally to stay in the room and promised to be right back, so we wouldn't miss the officers when they arrived. Sally said she would wait right there until I returned to be with her. In the meantime, the aide in the hallway would keep a close eye on Sally.

There was a local CVS Pharmacy nearby with COVID-19 tests, which had two tests inside. I headed back to the nursing home, intending to test Sally.

LaTisha and a police officer were standing just outside Sally's room when I arrived. LaTisha told the police officer that I was Sally's husband. Officer Raymond approached me and requested my statement. We agreed that after I checked on Sally, we would meet in the waiting area.

Sally was sitting right there in the chair watching TV like before. I told her I loved her and gave her a kiss. Yes, I kissed her even though she supposedly had COVID-19. Since she was feeling cold, I tucked her into her quilt, gave her another kiss, and assured her I'd be back in a few minutes following my conversation with Officer Raymond.

Sitting down, I told him the happenings of the night in question, and he recorded my statement to be transferred to this file that was being created on Helen. He asked if I was aware that Helen had been dismissed from her duties and that her employment at this place had ended.

No, I wasn't. LaTisha had given her the opportunity to resign, which she had done with no problems. His concern was that this nurse would show up at another facility and resume her cruel behavior towards residents. The existing laws prevented employers from stating resignation causes, thus Helen could seek opportunities in a different company.

"Officer, I'm just getting ready to test Sally. Would you watch and observe the results?" I asked.

He agreed. With protective clothing and a K95 mask, we walked into Sally's room.

"Sally, Baby, this is Officer Raymond. He's going to help us with the mean nurse problem."

She smiled and thanked him, telling him how scared she was of Helen.

"I need to test you for COVID-19."

"Ok," was her simple reply.

In just a couple of minutes, the test result was obvious—it was negative. The officer told me we needed to show the results to LaTisha.

We went to her office and were invited to come in. Handing her the test strip, the officer asked LaTisha if she had ever seen Sally's positive test. She stated that she had not; however, the test had been performed before her shift began.

The officer told her that Sally did not have COVID-19, and she agreed. We went to the on-site social worker and told her the results so that she could complete my wife's transfer to another facility. The social worker assured us she'd handle it and keep me informed.

Officer Raymond told me he would complete the investigation. He also told me the police department had many of these types of investigations, and not to hold my breath that the District Attorney's office would ever file charges against this nurse in question. The results of the investigation would be recorded and placed in a digital file. If any nursing home did a police check for potential issues with Helen, they would find this charge against her, along with others. He said he hoped more nursing homes would do complete investigations concerning potential caregivers, but that rarely happens. I thanked him for what he had done for us, and he left.

I RETURNED TO my wife's room. She was getting ready to eat lunch, so I sat down with her and helped. At about 1:30 p.m., after ensuring Sally was comfortable, I headed to the airport to pick up Johnna.

At about 3:00 p.m., Johnna and I returned to the facility and went to Sally's room. When we went in, she immediately spotted Johnna.

"Look who I found!" I said, delighted to see that Sally recognized her special visitor.

Some tears came to her eyes, tears of joy, and they hugged, kissed, and Sally told her how good it was to see her. Around 4:00 p.m., the social worker came in and told me to call Virginia at Focused Care, handing me her phone number.

Leaving Johnna with her mother, I stepped out of the room and headed to the lounge area to call Virginia. Immediately, she answered, informing me she was working on the ambulance transfer and was sure it would happen before noon the next day. She told me she would call back and give me all the details shortly. My wife would be in a safe place to live out the rest of her days!

Johnna informed me of her plan to stay with her mother overnight to ensure her safety. I dropped in on LaTisha to let her know what Johnna intended to do that evening. LaTisha said that given the circumstances, she'd make an exception to the policy preventing family members from staying overnight.

On my way back to the room, Virginia called, and the transfer was set. The people at Focused Care were expecting Sally shortly after noon the next day. I informed Johnna that her overnight stay was approved, and she could use the other bed. The cafeteria staff was even going to bring an extra dinner for Johnna when they brought Sally's meal to her. So, everyone was taken care of for the evening, but me! Johnna just had to be on guard until noon the next day.

We were totally relieved! Even Sally seemed to be eager about the move to a new place. But first, we prayed and thanked our Lord for getting us through this difficult time and for the pending transfer, also for making this transfer a very smooth, enjoyable event.

Shortly after eating, we packed up all of Sally's things in her large plastic tubs and laid out her clothes for the next day. During this time, she was very upbeat, eyes sparkling, and she was smiling her tremendously infectious smile. Sally was happy for a change.

Glimpse: Her eyes sparkled, and she smiled with her tremendously infectious smile.

TWELVE

A Safe Place

*The world can only seem a safe place
when we feel safe inside.*
AGAPI STASSINOPOULOS

The next day, it seemed like it took forever for the transfer ambulance to arrive. The people from the ambulance service called me at about 10:00 a.m. and told me the transfer ambulance would be there at about noon. They asked if Sally had a wheelchair. She did not, so they told me not to be concerned because they had plenty and would bring one for her. After this call, it seemed like time sped up. Johnna and Sally's lunch was brought to the room, and I pulled mine out of my lunch bag.

After lunch, the transfer ambulance arrived right on time. The attendant came in with the wheelchair, told us her name (Sue), and that she would take care of Sally. She asked if one of us wanted to ride in the front of the ambulance, to which Johnna said she would. The trip would take a little over one hour to get to Focused Care. Sally was strapped into the rear of the ambulance in a wheelchair. She was not thrilled about this, but she relaxed when she found out that Johnna would ride with her. Following the ambulance in my truck, we would all arrive at the same time.

When we arrived, Sue went to work getting Sally unbuckled and out of the ambulance. A little smile came to her face, and she asked if this was her new home. She smiled when I told her this was her new temporary home and that she would be well cared for here.

When we entered Focused Care, the social worker, Liz, met us at the door, and we followed her to Sally's room. She had a roommate who was there recuperating from hip surgery and who was experiencing dementia. People came to her room and completed the check-in so that everything was taken care of in a warm, family-like setting—totally different from the other facility. Everything was explained, including meals and where they would be given, bathing, and her scheduled days and time for that to take place. All this seemed to flow so well. I could tell she was feeling more and more comfortable.

I was asked about Sally and her Sundowner's Syndrome. They told me not to worry as they would take care of her. They *did* want to place a warning ankle bracelet on her, just in case she would try to go out one of the doors. They all had alarms on them that would be triggered by the ankle bracelet. We agreed to this. The ankle bracelet was red, white, and blue, so Sally really liked it. I think she thought of it as a piece of jewelry. Heading to the finance office to pay her co-pay for March, the people in the finance office had talked to Jennifer, our estate planning attorney, concerning the Medicaid application and where that process was. All was well.

Johnna, Sally, and I decided to go for a walk around the facility and find out where things were located. All the staff came and called her by name and told her that if she needed anything to just ask one of them and they would help her with any request. What a difference the personnel were at this facility; it seemed like they wanted to care for her.

We were served dinner with her that evening and were asked afterward if we would be there for breakfast. We told them we would not, but we would be there after breakfast. We took her back to her room, got her PJs on, turned her TV on, and she settled into bed. It was not too long before she told us she was tired. She had been through a big day, and she needed to sleep.

We told her we loved her, hugged her, gave her kisses, and left. She was asleep, I think, before we left the room. Johnna and I headed home, and we talked about how relieved we were that we now had Sally in a safe place.

SUNDOWNER'S SYNDROME

Observations: This is a common behavior in someone with Alzheimer's or dementia. Symptoms like anxiety, hallucinations, and confusion appear later in the day, coinciding with sunset. Though delirium can arise at any point, it typically manifests most frequently as the day progresses. As evening approaches and the light fades, you might observe your loved one engaged in repetitive actions (see the following symptoms).

- Pacing
- Fidgeting
- Wandering
- Anger and agitation
- Crying
- Paranoia
- Mental states of confusion, including irritation and hallucinations

Healthcare providers cite interrupted sleep patterns and medication side effects as potential causes for this. But other factors like low lighting, overstimulation from a busy day, and pain or physical illness can also be triggers for the behaviors associated with Sundowner's Syndrome.

What You Can Do: When your loved one's demeanor shifts toward the end of the day, assist them in calming down by implementing these strategies:

- Keep their environment quiet and free from electronics and television.

[cont'd next page]

-Use white noise or soft music to soothe their soul.
-Read to them.
-Follow the same routine, at the same time, when preparing for bed (e.g., wash face, comb hair, put on pajamas, take medicine, turn off lights, etc.).
-Avoid eating food, alcohol, or snacks within three hours of bedtime (unless evening medication requires something light, such as a cracker).
-Help them get plenty of sunlight during the day and minimize naps too late in the day.

AT ABOUT 9:00 A.M. the next day, we found Sally outside her room. She was inside the nurses' station with a stack of papers. Seeing us, she approached us with a huge smile and lively eyes.

"I've been helping the nurses while waiting for you," she said, hugging Johnna.

After what she had been through—what *we* had been through together—I finally felt confident that we had her in the right place.

Glimpse: She greeted them with a huge smile, lively eyes, and was busy "helping" the nurses.

As we went to the dining room to grab a cup of coffee and visit, I was amazed by how comfortable and less reserved Sally was. At the beginning, she was constantly on edge, always moving closer to me when the staff talked to her or were just walking by.

Midway through our visit, Aymie, the director of nurses at Focused Care, walked over and asked if I had a moment to talk in her office. Leaving Sally with Johnna, I made my way to the office and sat down. I'll admit, I was slightly on the defensive, ready to protect my wife over whatever problem called for this meeting. She began by telling me how sweet and loving Sally was. So far, so good. But I knew there was going to be more, so I just continued to listen.

"The problem is, she gets out of bed at about 10:00 p.m. and walks the halls, usually winding up at the nurses' station."

Upon further explanation, I learned that the nurse working the night shift talked to Sally about why she was awake that late. The recorded response was that she just woke up and wanted to see if she could assist with anything. The nurse immediately gave her a task, one that did not mean anything to anyone except Sally.

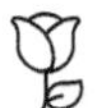 **Glimpse:** She wanted to help the nurses at the nurses' station.

After about two hours, the job was done, and she was ready to sleep. The nurse walked Sally to her room, making sure she lay in bed, before returning to the nurses' station. And thankfully, she stayed asleep until being awoken for her shower the next morning.

Apparently, that type of behavior was not uncommon. We both hoped that with time, Sally could relax enough to start falling asleep more easily at night. If not, Aymie told me that the night nurse would give her something to do, and she could just stay at the nurses' station.

"The night nurses rarely have much to do, and that shift could be rather boring, so having someone to talk to is a plus and makes their shift go by much faster," Aymie reassured me, relieving my stress in that moment. This facility was a totally different type of care than she had received at the previous one. I felt far more comfortable with my wife in their care.

Aymie also informed me about an instance with Sally one night when she was working the night shift as the nurse in charge. Sally had walked out of her room and down the hall to the nurses' station. It was about 11:00 p.m., when all the residents were asleep except for some in the isolation hall.

This hall has a one-way door that can be opened from the outside, so a person can enter the hallway but needs an employee badge to go back through. Sally was there in the nurses' station with Aymie, organizing some papers. She noticed a lady trying to get through the locked door.

One thing about my wife that never changed, even throughout her battle with dementia/Alzheimer's, was that she was always ready to help anyone. Sally would often ask people, even total strangers, "Are you doing all right?" Unlike most people who might ask you that same question, she really wanted to know if you were all right. If you needed something or if you needed help, she would do whatever she could to help you or get what you needed.

Glimpse: She was always ready to help anyone and genuinely cared if they were all right.

Many times, we would be in the checkout line at the grocery store, and Sally would start talking to the person in line behind us. She would finally ask if they were all right or if they needed help. Often, this person in line, whom she did not know, would tell her about their current circumstances.

I can't remember how many times Sally would tell me that the person behind us in line needed help paying for their groceries. Then she would ask, "Do you think we can help them?" We would wait until their groceries were totaled, and then I would pay for their groceries. She was just naturally that way, always striving to be kind and generous to someone who might need a little help.

Glimpse: Sally was always striving to be kind and generous to those who might need help.

The moment Sally noticed the woman on the other side of the door, she got up from her seat in the nurses' station and walked out of the nurses' station. She was about to push the door open when Aymie hollered at her to stop. Aymie told her she could not open that locked door. Unaware that she was doing anything wrong, she told her she was only trying to help that nice lady get through the door.

When Aymie told me this story, I looked at her and said, "That's my baby, always trying to help someone." Aymie agreed, and we both laughed!

THINGS WENT ALONG fine, and in about a week, Johnna had to leave and get back home to Wichita, Kansas, so that she could do her work from her home computer. She told her mother the next day that she was going to be gone for a little while, but she would come back to see her. Sally was fine with that. They said goodbye, and I drove Johnna to the airport. I let Sally know I'd be back later that day, after she ate lunch.

Time meant little to Sally anymore. She was at the point in her dementia/Alzheimer's that she lost her sense of time. To her, the day was dictated by showers, meals, activities, and then bedtime. She was becoming more relaxed, but some members of the staff still made her nervous. I really felt it was because she had little to no daily contact with them.

The next day, I arrived at about 8:00 a.m. and joined Sally in the dining hall, where she was finishing her breakfast. Vanessa, the activities director, came in and sat down with us at the table.

"So, what does Sally like to do in her free time?" she asked.

"She likes music, especially church hymns, coloring, and Bible study. Is there a regular Bible study for the residents?"

"We used to have a pastor who would come once a week, but he stopped. I've been hosting them myself, but don't feel the most qualified."

Being a pastor, I saw this as a perfect opportunity to step in and potentially lead the weekly Bible study, which would allow me to both spread God's word and spend more time with my wife. However, I had never held a Bible study in a place where most of the residents had memory issues. "Would it be okay if I sat in on the next study to observe how it's run?" I asked Vanessa.

"Of course! They're held every Tuesday at 10:00 a.m.," she said eagerly.

The next Tuesday came, and I arrived at about 8:30 a.m. Sally was watching TV in her room. I told her I loved her and gave her a kiss. She did the same.

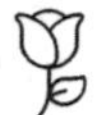 **Glimpse:** She told me she loved me and gave me a kiss.

The day was starting well. We went to the entryway and sat on the couch together. On the way, I noticed a member of the staff, someone I had not seen before, come by, and Sally went into her shell and moved close to me.

One nurse, Jennifer, noticed this, and she came up to Sally and me, put her arms around her, and told her that everyone there loved her and would do nothing that would cause her any problems. Sally became so happy, her eyes sparkled, she put on her huge, beautiful smile, and she told Vanessa she loved her. That was the day that she no longer showed any form of fear or caution concerning any of the staff.

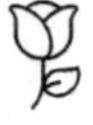 **Glimpse:** Her eyes sparkled, and she put on her huge, beautiful smile.

It was almost time for the Bible study, and we spotted Vanessa gathering the residents. We went to the dining hall and took our seats as the other residents who needed help were brought in. Just a few minutes before 10:00 a.m., Vanessa started things off with some sing-along hymns on a

YouTube channel. Everyone joined in the singing, and Sally was having a wonderful time.

After about three or four songs, Vanessa stepped up and spoke. I was excited to see how she would work with the residents. Instead, she introduced me as Sally's husband and a pastor, who would start leading them in the Bible study. So much for watching and learning! It was now my responsibility to lead these residents in the Bible study.

Since the twenty or so residents there knew little about me, I started by giving a brief introduction about myself and my experience in serving two churches on Sundays.

"Is there anything you all would like me to do during the Bible study time, aside from teaching about the Bible?" I asked, attempting to find the most effective way to run these studies.

There was no response. Asking direct questions would not work. The most productive route would be to take over and tell them what we were going to do.

So, that morning, I explained that the Bible was a love story—a story about how much God, our Father in Heaven, loved us. I shared all the things he did for the ancient people, especially his chosen Israelite nation, and how he sent Moses to lead them out of captivity. After a brief discussion, I told them I'd be back next Tuesday, and we would start with the Book of Matthew in the New Testament. The intent would be to go verse by verse and discuss the meaning within each group of Scriptures.

One lady spoke up and asked, "Are you going to bring treats?"

I replied to that question with, "What kind would you like?" She responded that they really didn't care as long as there were plenty of them. The session was then closed with prayer, and Vanessa came back up. We sang a couple more hymns before we were dismissed.

This special time ultimately became a regular part of my life, and I was blessed to go to Focused Care every Tuesday and lead this Bible study for the residents. I was also part of a men's Bible study in my subdivision every Tuesday morning from 8:00–9:30 a.m. Since Focused Care was only about a 10-minute drive, I had no problem doing both. Tuesday mornings were busy for me, but it was a blessing to prepare for both equally important Bible studies.

Every Tuesday at Focused Care started with going straight to Sally's room with my handful of stuff for the Bible study. She would always look at me and put her hand on my Bible with sparkling eyes as she would ask, "Are you going to teach the 'peoples'?"

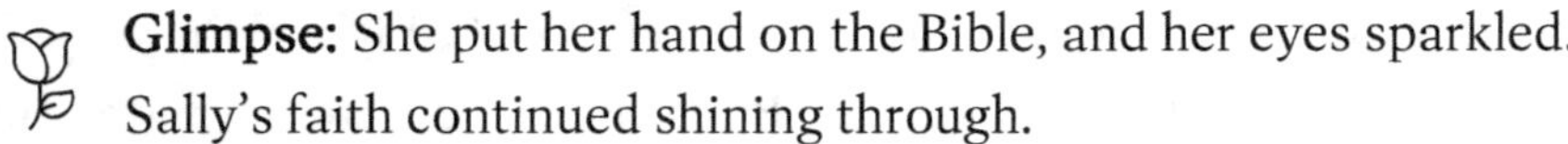 **Glimpse:** She put her hand on the Bible, and her eyes sparkled. Sally's faith continued shining through.

She referred to all the Bible study attendees as "the peoples," because she could not remember any of their names.

Early on, she would come and sit in a chair in the dining hall during the Bible study. She would always be in the front row. I remember the many times during teaching the "peoples," looking over to where she was sitting and seeing that sparkle in her eyes and that smile on her face. She felt happy and proud. This study continued every Tuesday.

Once Sally graduated from this life to her eternal life, I continued that study every Tuesday for almost one full year.

Glimpse: The sparkle in her eyes and her big smile continued during every Bible study until Sally went to her eternal home.

THIRTEEN

Hospice

The end of life deserves as much beauty, care,
and respect as the beginning.

ANONYMOUS

One morning at the facility, Jennifer asked me if I had considered getting hospice involved in Sally's care. As a pastor, my dealings with hospice agencies and their very qualified people were normally right at the very end of a person's life. She told me that was one function of hospice, but now, before a person gets to that point, hospice has what is called "interim care."

She explained that, if I chose that service, then Sally would get an additional RN to visit her on regular visits to monitor her condition. She would also receive an aide who would come three times a week to bathe, dress, and monitor Sally's health. She would also get a chaplain who would visit regularly, at least once a week. They would spend time with her doing different things and would pray for and with her if she desired.

We would also have a dedicated social worker to monitor her case and the progression of the dementia/Alzheimer's. She would meet with me regularly. There would be a monthly conference with the social worker and the RN to keep me apprised of what was happening and what to expect. In addition, Sally would get a doctor who would see her at least monthly, but more often if directed by the RN or social worker. All these people would be in control of Sally's treatment and care.

As I thought about this, there did not seem to be any downside to my wife's treatment. Would she recommend a hospice service? She explained that there were several who worked with residents at Focused Care. She reached over to the nurses' station and handed me a brochure from Oasis Hospice. I contacted them and set up a meeting to talk about their care and what it would entail.

Accepting the Inevitable

As Alzheimer's patients visibly deteriorate, the prospect of their eventual death becomes undeniable. Accepting the inevitable is not easy, but you've already made a good start by picking up this book. The first thing to remember is: you're not alone.

There are support groups, hospice groups, and mentors who can walk with you through that journey. They may advise you to document the everyday and special moments, have important conversations, share memories, find a supportive community, and try to remain present.

While anticipatory grief may bring out anger or resentment, it can also equip you against regret. Express your emotions honestly (if perhaps privately) and allow your loved one to do so as well.

As Alzheimer's alters relationships, allow yourself to grieve the person you've lost over the course of the disease. Remember, experiencing grief and attempting to heal is not a linear process.

The next day, the social worker who worked at Focused Care met with me. She basically repeated what Vanessa had already told me. My insurance covered their service, so there would be no additional cost for Sally's care. I agreed to use their service, and the next day, we met the RN who would attend to Sally. Her name was Gloria, the same name as the caregiver from Pam's Senior Helpers. It was a different person, but I felt like my Lord had just given me a sign that everything was going to be all right. After signing all the paperwork, we were on our way to getting my wife additional people to care for her.

The next day, I arrived and met with the new people from Oasis Hospice, along with staff from Focused Care. Jennifer went through everything again, and Dr. Patel, from Oasis Hospice, told me he had looked at Sally's medication list and he had a few questions.

"How often does Sally experience uncontrolled anxiety?"

"Rarely. I'm almost always able to calm her down," I assured him.

"What would happen if you were not there?"

There was no way for me to answer that question because I didn't know what would happen. Dr. Patel could sense my uncertainty and told me both he and Gloria were going to work with the staff nurses and see if any adjustments in her one medication were warranted. He gave me his business card and told me not to hesitate to text him with questions. He assured me he would respond within the hour, as long as it was not before 6:00 a.m. or after 8:00 p.m.

Seeing my discomfort, Gloria chimed in. "While we're here to help Sally, we're also here to help you through this difficult time. We will always advise you on the many upcoming decisions that involve you as Sally's medical and financial power of attorney."

Gloria would begin seeing Sally on Tuesday and Friday for the first four weeks at 11:00 a.m. She told me she was aware of the Bible study at 10:00 a.m., and she did not want to interfere with that. Her part would only take 15 to 20 minutes, so it would also not interfere with lunch. I felt very good about this. We all headed for Sally's room together.

When we arrived at her room, she looked at me and the other three from Oasis with a bit of a confused look. I greeted her as I always did, expressing my love with a kiss and a big hug. After being introduced to the Oasis Hospice crew, she smiled and told us she felt really special to have all these people caring for her.

Everyone responded that she was indeed unique! Gloria went about doing the exam, which included blood pressure, heart rate, breathing rate, and listening to her lungs and heart. All seemed well, and Sally enjoyed the attention. I could tell that Gloria was a real hit with her, especially when she asked if she could get a big hug.

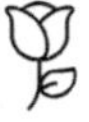 **Glimpse:** Sally was a person who loved to give and receive hugs.

This care given by hospice was tremendous, and the next day I met Sherri, the aide who would bathe Sally three times a week or more, if required. Sally was a challenge to bathe (believe me, I know from personal experience), but it turned out that Sherri did not seem to have any issues with her at all. Sally really liked Sherri, so bathing became something she looked forward to. Sherri would also rub lotion all over her body to keep her skin soft and very elastic. The largest organ we have is the skin, and we need to care for it.

Like Sally, I looked forward to the visits by Gloria, Sherri, Jennifer, and Allen, the chaplain. They were there, primarily for Sally, but also to care for me during the transition as her illness progressed. I did not look forward to those times or those dramatic decisions. Still, because of my study and reading about this disease, I anticipated them. And these decisions concerning my wife and her care, and ultimately her life, would be left up to me.

FOURTEEN

Conversations

*A ten-minute conversation with the person you love
is enough to keep you happy all day long.*
ANONYMOUS

Throughout our married life, which lasted just over 50 years, we were as close as any married couple I had ever witnessed. Throughout my time in ministry, I had witnessed several married couples who were probably just as close to being one as we were, but there were few.

Most couples that society would classify as successful couples have their differences. These differences can grow and become a real problem if the couple in question does not do everything they can to minimize those differences. We had some early in our marriage. After all, we were two individual persons with our own ideas of how things should be and how we should act toward one another as husband and wife.

Before placing Sally in a skilled nursing facility, Johnna and I (mainly Johnna) bought picture albums, and Johnna organized pictures inside them and labeled them. Some of these people I did not know well, so that really came in handy when we went through them together. There were pictures in one album of all the grandchildren at different ages. In the other album were pictures of family, aunts, uncles, children, mothers, fathers, and some pictures of the vacation trips we had made together.

 **Glimpse:** Family was very important to Sally. Looking at the albums allowed her to remember and connect with their love.

Now, every week, I would sit with her to flip through the picture albums, telling her who the individuals pictured were. When we looked at these pictures, and she saw someone who was extra special, she would take her right hand and touch that picture. She would normally always touch the head of the person, indicating that she knew that person was special to her.

With her illness, I could tell by looking at the pictures with her what place that person held in her memory. All of them would be classed as long-term memory so that she would know, or I thought she knew, who they were.

One album at a time, we would look through it. I noticed that as the illness worsened, her reaction to certain pictures seemed to change. A picture that was a special memory one week was erased the next. There was no way for me to understand the reason for this. I noticed the change over time and knew this was all part of the disease. The disease would ultimately take her life. There was absolutely no cure. When we finished looking at an album, she would always smile and always tell me, "Everything is going to be all right."

Glimpse: Sally continued to reassure others, "Everything is going to be all right."

DURING THE FIRST few months at Focused Care, she seemed to improve mentally. I believe this happened because she felt safe and comfortable there with the staff and the other residents with whom she interacted daily. She became a little more vocal and could carry on a conversation with full sentences. I knew this wouldn't last and wasn't ready for it to end.

During this time, we had many conversations about essentially everything. Some things were about her and me, some things about life, and some spiritual things. I remember one morning, she told me she needed to tell me something.

"I saw the angels, and they scared me. There weren't many, but I didn't recognize any of them."

I wasn't exactly sure how to respond to this statement. But I gave her a comforting look and said, "If they were truly angels, sent by the Lord, there's no reason to be scared by their visit."

From my time in the ministry dealing with those who are close to the end of their time on earth, I knew that this was normally a precursor of things to come. The only thing that concerned me was her being frightened by the angels. I knew where my wife was in her faith and especially her relationship with her Lord Jesus Christ. So, I just placed this in the back of my mind, hoping she would tell me more later.

ON ANOTHER DAY, she looked at me with troubled eyes. I asked her if she was all right, and she instantly responded, "I am all right."

But then she looked straight at me, analyzing my facial expression.

"Are *you* all right?" she asked with a puzzled look.

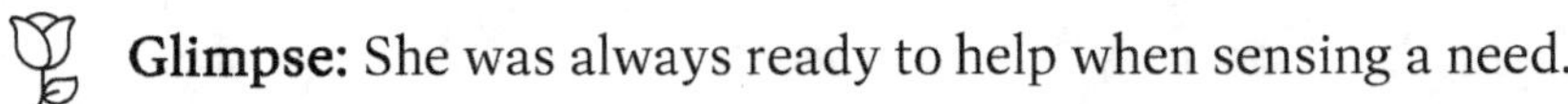 **Glimpse:** She was always ready to help when sensing a need.

She knew when something was on my mind or if I was going through some troubling time. "Yes, but we're just having some trouble finding enough volunteers for the Lord's Pantry at church."

We operated a food pantry with one of the other churches in Leona. I had started announcing from the pulpit on Sunday mornings, before the start of the worship service, that we needed more volunteers for those Thursday mornings. Barbara was now heading the volunteers and their scheduling. The current problem was that she just had enough volunteers for one Thursday, so these volunteers would work every Thursday that our churches worked the pantry. She told me not to worry about the need for more volunteers because "the Lord would supply them."

"We need to pray about the volunteers we currently have and for the new ones that are to come forward and volunteer," Sally insisted.

We joined hands and began by thanking the Lord for all those who were currently volunteering. We asked for blessings for each one of them. We asked the Lord to touch people within our congregation and bring them to Barbara so she would have more than enough people to take care of working each Thursday. We closed the prayer by again thanking the Lord for bringing those additional people forward as volunteers.

At the end of the prayer, she told me not to worry anymore because it had been taken care of by our Lord, and Barbara would have plenty of volunteers! She has taught me over the years, again and again, to go to the Lord first, and He will take care of the little things—and I'm still learning this lesson.

She reminded me of what Jesus said in Matthew 9:37b-38:

> *The harvest is great, but the workers are few.*
> *So pray to the Lord who is in charge of the harvest;*
> *ask him to send more workers into his fields.*
> MATTHEW 9:37B-38 (NLT)

Hearing her quoting scripture again was music to my ears, because it had been a while since she could remember the loads of scriptures she had stored within her mind. As mentioned earlier, I felt she was showing a moment in time when she was mentally better, and it was comforting to know that she was relaxed and felt safe in this place.

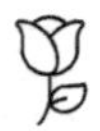 **Glimpse:** Her faith continued to shine through the disease of Alzheimer's.

The following Sunday, when I stepped up to the pulpit to make the announcement concerning volunteers for the "Lord's Pantry," Barbara stopped me at the first of the announcement and said she now had a group of volunteers, but she would always welcome more. I smiled and immediately remembered what my baby had told me after we had prayed, asking the Lord for more volunteers.

The congregation probably wondered why I had such a huge smile on my face, but I knew that our prayer had been answered. My mind immediately ran to James 5:16b (NLT), which states, "The earnest prayer of a righteous person has great power and produces wonderful results."

My wife was truly a righteous person, and she was doing her best to get me to that point in my life. It was working because her faith demonstrated her righteous power, and it also showed that I, too, could have that power from the Lord.

A FEW WEEKS went by. Sally could still talk and carry on a reasonable conversation. She agreed to spend some time with me to look through another photo album, one full of pictures of our family. We carried the photo album to the front lounge area and snuggled up beside each other on the couch. There was no one else in the front lounge area that morning—just Sally and me.

The first picture was a photo of her mother and father. She took her hand, placed it on the picture, and looked up at me with tearful eyes.

"They are not there," she sighed with a hurt voice.

I could tell this was an emotional thing for her, so I told her it was all right. But she spoke in a more forceful tone, "I told you they are not there."

Not really knowing what she meant and not wanting to upset her any more than she already was, I just turned the page.

The next picture was one of her and me when we re-did our wedding vows on our 25th wedding anniversary. She again placed her hand on the picture and looked at me. But this time her eyes were sparkling, no tears in sight.

"I'm going to be all right, and you are going to be all right."

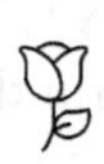 **Glimpse:** Sally was always reassuring others she was going to be all right, but she also reassured John that *he* was going to be all right. This time, her comment was related to spiritual insight.

It was good to see the change in her, but I still couldn't get over the statement concerning her parents not being there. I was not sure what she meant by "not there." The first thing that came to my mind was the statement she had made to me concerning the angels coming to her, and that it scared her. But it could mean a lot of things; I just had no way of knowing exactly.

We continued that morning, looking through the family album. When different family members came up in the pictures, she would touch those pictures, and then she would smile. Then one of Sally's aides came over to let her know lunch was about to be served.

"Perfect timing. We just finished going through this photo album." I directed my attention back to Sally. "I need to leave for a little while, but will be back shortly. Enjoy your lunch. I love you."

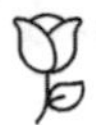 **Glimpse:** When I looked at her, she gave me a big smile and wanted a kiss.

A WEEK WENT by, and we were having another conversation. Sally brought up the angels again. This time, she told me that when the angels came to visit her so she was not scared anymore. I asked her if Jesus was with them, and she told me He was not, but the angels told her He would come to her later. Now things were making sense concerning the angels.

In my time in the ministry, I have had many people, ones with a really close relationship with the Lord, tell me they knew Jesus was coming to get them. In John 14:3, Jesus tells us,

> *When everything is ready, I will come and get you,*
> *so that you will always be with me where I am.*
> JOHN 14:3 (NLT)

She told me she knew he was coming for her, but "everything" must be ready. I have often wondered if she had actually experienced a glimpse of heaven and the people there because of these visits from the angels. One can only imagine what she had seen and experienced.

A FUN CONVERSATION with Sally always involved Dairy Queen ice cream. She loved ice cream, so frequently when I would return in the afternoon, I would stop by the local Dairy Queen and get her a small cup of ice cream, along with one for her roommate and, of course, myself. One thing about Sally and her ice cream is that it was hers and hers alone—no sharing!

On the occasions when I would get Sally and her roommate a small cup of ice cream, if I asked her if I could have a bite, she would tell me, "NO!" Because of that, I always purchased one for myself. The ice cream was something that, even after she had started being fed by the staff, had no problem eating by herself. She would take that spoon and that cup of ice cream, and eat every bit, with no help whatsoever!

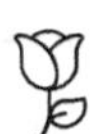 **Glimpse:** She savored her Dairy Queen ice cream and refused to share any of it!

Having Conversations

These strategies may be helpful in communicating with your loved one:

- Give the loved one time to process what you have said. Allow them a moment to form a response.
- Reduce distractions, including noise and other conversations.
- Speak clearly; avoid mumbling or covering your face with your hands when talking. Keep the language simple.
- Communicate good listening skills by nodding, using eye contact, and friendly expressions. If they are in a wheelchair, you may need to sit down to converse with them at eye level.
- Join the journey. Participate in their train of thought rather than accusing or resisting, as long as there are no safety issues.
- When bringing up memories, say "*I* remember when ...." Don't ask them if *they* remember when ....
- Don't talk about them in front of others; include them in the conversation.
- Provide reassurance. Reassure them that they are not the problem. Say, "We're going to figure this out together," or "I'll do a better job communicating with you."
- Speak to them as adults while practicing patience. Avoid arguing.
- Focus on the present moment when starting a conversation. "Are you?" vs. "Did you?"
- Notice phrases, cues, or people they respond well to. Utilize those when possible.
- Redirect to something that is calming or holds their interest if they do not understand your conversation. Activities such as eating, looking at familiar photos, singing a song, or doing an activity together may be comforting ways to redirect.

FIFTEEN

A Special Visit

Other things may change us,
but we start and end with the family.
ANTHONY BRANDT

The dementia/Alzheimer's was progressing. Sally was having a really difficult time walking because the disease was affecting her equilibrium. The only way she could walk down the halls was to use the handrails on both sides of the hall. When she got to the end of the handrail and tried to go on, she would fall.

The nurse in charge called me one day at about 2:00 p.m. to tell me it had happened again, only this time, she had hit her head on the floor. Thankfully, she didn't have any significant problems. Nevertheless, they had contacted Gloria, the hospice RN, and she was on her way to check on her.

When I arrived at Focused Care, she had a slight bump on her head. Gloria was there and informed me that there weren't any issues. She had used her light and checked both eyes and found no difference in the reaction of the pupil from one eye to the other. Sally was responsive, or as responsive as she could be. Gloria and I put Sally in bed. "Do you want to take a little nap?" I asked. She looked at me and just nodded, then closed her eyes and went to sleep.

Gloria and I discussed the fall and the minor blow to her head. Because of what she had seen looking in her eyes and her verbal responses to the questions, she did not feel like there was a problem.

"Since the dementia/Alzheimer's is progressing and her brain is dying slowly, do you think there was no trauma to the brain because of the added space between her brain and the skull?" I asked Gloria.

"That is definitely a possibility," she responded.

Sally's nap lasted maybe an hour. When she woke up, I was there to hold her and tell her I loved her. She smiled and told me she knew that—some of the greatest words I've ever heard.

Glimpse: She smiled and said she knew he loved her—a familiar response.

I told her that our daughter, Tonya, and granddaughter, Maggie, were flying in the next day to see her. She was delighted, and her eyes sparkled as she said, "That will be nice."

Glimpse: Her eyes sparkled, and Sally said, "That will be nice."

The next day, I prepared to leave at lunchtime. Let me explain why I did not stay around when it was time for Sally to eat a meal. If I were there, Sally would tell me she was full after only a very few bites, and I wouldn't try to force her to eat more.

If the staff personnel were feeding her, they would play a little game with her, telling her she had promised to take one more bite. They would tell her, "one more bite," until she had eaten everything on her plate. I had to learn not to be there during meals because she would stop eating, no matter who was feeding her. Sally actually gained weight—not much, four pounds—but at this time, that was a lot of weight for her to gain.

The time came for Sally to go to lunch. I told her I'd be back in a little while after I picked up Tonya and Maggie from Houston Intercontinental Airport (now called George Bush Intercontinental Airport).

As described earlier, our visit with them on Thanksgiving resulted in losing Sally at a Love's fuel stop on the way home. Because of that, we no longer traveled. Maggie and Sally had really bonded on that trip, so I was excited to see Maggie and Tonya. Tonya had told Maggie about how much Sally had changed mentally, so she understood that her grandmother might not recognize her. But not to worry—take it one day at a time.

I picked them up at the airport with no issues. The plane was on time, and all baggage arrived with them, so we loaded up in my truck and headed for Huntsville. Since they had been traveling most of the morning, I inquired if they were hungry. Asking a 16-year-old girl if she is hungry when she has had nothing to eat in over four hours is not my smartest question. Of course, they were hungry!

We stopped at a restaurant nearby that served a variety of things to eat and placed our orders. Maggie asked me how her grandmother was doing. She also wanted to know if she could recognize people, especially family. Most mornings, she could recognize who people were, including family, but during the afternoon, she seemed to lose some of that capability.

We finished our meal, loaded back into the truck, and continued to head for the nursing home. When we arrived and got out of the truck, as we went inside, I took Maggie by the hand and told her to walk with me. We walked, hand in hand, down the hallway toward Grandma's room. When we entered her room, she was snoozing—not fully asleep but just on the verge of a nap.

As we entered the room, with me still holding Maggie's hand, I said, "Sally, it's John. Look who I found! Someone has come to see you!" When I called her name, she opened her eyes and immediately spotted Maggie. She came to life, eyes sparkled, big smile, her hands extended, ready to give Maggie a hug. As she hugged Maggie, she spotted Tonya and lifted one hand to her.

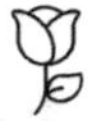 **Glimpse:** Her eyes sparkled, she gave a big smile, and Sally's hands extended, ready for a hug.

This family gathering could not have been better. Maggie and Tonya sat on her bed, and they started talking. Sally responded with short sentences. I could see relief come over our granddaughter's face, and her body relaxed. All the worry and tension about how her grandma would react to her quickly dissipated and was replaced with joy.

Maggie did a great job talking to her grandma. I mean that she did not ask a bunch of questions, but would tell her she remembered when Sally and I came to visit them over Thanksgiving in Mesa, Arizona. She talked about the things she did with her grandma and how happy that visit made her feel. She told her grandma that during that visit, she had made her feel important. That was one of the many things that Sally had the ability and character to make people feel. They were the center of her attention, and they were very important.

Tonya continued to sit on the bed with her, and she started telling Sally about all the things going on with all the kids. She told her about Maggie making it to the "Brown Level" of the Centurion Krav Maga, a self-defense system. She was the youngest person, at 16 years old, to accomplish this level. She told her about Emily and her decision to change her career pathway. She was now going to get her real estate license and go to work in that industry. It seemed to always be busy with so many people moving to Arizona and looking for homes.

She talked about Jack and how he wanted to go into the IT industry to study computer technology. He had visited the Microsoft facility there in the Phoenix area and talked to some of their recruiters. He had hoped to get a position with them as an intern while he pursued his education in computer technology. But he was disappointed when he was told Microsoft was changing its position and looking for more people involved in artificial intelligence instead of computer technology. At least the people at Microsoft hadn't misled him. He was in limbo as to what he would pursue now and was investigating other options.

Maggie, of course, was still in high school but was looking into the future possibility of becoming an EMT. I could tell Sally was taking all this in and really enjoying the time with Tonya and Maggie.

She looked at me and asked if we still had the funds, meaning 529 college funds, for the kids. I told her that Emily had already received hers and that it took care of her associate's degree. But we still had them for Jack and for Maggie. When they needed them, Tonya would let me know, and they would receive those funds as their needs warranted. She smiled her big, beautiful smile, then she told us she was tired.

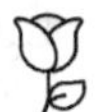 **Glimpse:** She smiled with her big, beautiful smile.

Maggie helped her get into bed for an early afternoon nap before dinner, and she went right to sleep. We left and headed for home so they could unload their suitcases and get settled in for our dinner together.

THE NEXT COUPLE of days went well, with Sally enjoying the time with Tonya and Maggie. On the third day, in the afternoon, Maggie noticed that her grandma was not very perky and was not really responding to much of anything.

She also noticed her eyes and how they seemed lifeless. I tried to explain that her eyes had become my measuring stick to determine how alert she was. If her eyes were sparkling, then she was alert and cognizant. If her eyes were like what I termed "doll's eyes" and lifeless, she was awake, but nothing was really happening.

I thought about those times when the lights were on, but no one was home. Those were the times when I felt like she knew I was there, and she was comfortable with that. But she was in a different realm mentally and was not really cognizant of what was going on or who was there.

She knew we were there, but she possibly did not know who we were. Maggie indicated that she understood the circumstances and that this was just part of the horrible disease.

DOLL'S EYES IN AN ALZHEIMER'S PATIENT

When Alzheimer's patients have *"doll's eyes"* (also known as a positive oculocephalic reflex), this indicates that the cerebral cortex is damaged or disconnected from the brainstem. It's a neurodegenerative illness where the VOR (vestibular-ocular reflex) is not controlled, leading the eyes to fixate straight ahead instead of tracking moving objects when the head is in motion.

In a healthy person, the eyes move independently of head movement. In advanced Alzheimer's, this inhibition is lost, and the brainstem takes over, making the eyes appear lifeless or like a doll's eyes.

IT CAME TIME for Tonya and Maggie to return to their home in Arizona. Their flight left Houston at 3:00 p.m., so I needed to have them at the airport by at least 2:00 p.m. We went to visit Sally for the last time, and I told them not to say goodbye but to tell her they were going to leave for a little while, but they would see her again.

With this disease, time meant nothing to Sally, especially since it was in an advanced stage. She only understood time as it related to her schedule—when she was taken by a nurse or an aide to do something.

For her, it may be time to bathe, or it was time for breakfast, lunch, or dinner. It was time to go to sleep. Nothing in her day was related to time according to a clock.

The morning visit went very well, with Sally being bright-eyed and able to communicate with one-word or very few-word sentences. Just about 11:30 a.m., one aide, Jessica, came to see if Sally wanted her lunch brought to her or if she wanted to go to the dining hall to eat. She indicated she wanted to go to the dining hall, so Jessica started getting her out of bed and into her wheelchair. We told her we were going to leave for a little while, gave her hugs and kisses, and left just as Jessica took her and headed to lunch.

We went and loaded up into the truck, and off we headed to the airport, stopping off for something to eat first. Maggie talked about her visit with her grandma and how she could never forget the time she had with her. She was elated that she could come with her mother to see Grandma and Grandpa. I could tell she was relieved that her grandma recognized her during the visit, with just a couple of afternoons when she had doll eyes.

We ate lunch at a place relatively close to the airport and then proceeded to the airport drop-off point. Before I left them, we prayed together, shed a tear or three, and they went inside the airport for their flight home. It was on time, which meant they would get home at about 4:00 p.m. because of the two-hour time difference. I headed back to Huntsville and home and planned to return to the nursing home after the evening meal, where I would stay until Sally went to sleep.

SIXTEEN

The Disease Worsens

While no one can change the outcome of dementia
or Alzheimer's, with the right support
you can change the journey.
TARA REED

Over the next several days, Sally's health declined, with fewer periods of alertness. Gloria, the RN in charge of Sally's case at Oasis Hospice, led the meeting after she checked Sally's vital signs. When Oasis Hospice first started their care of Sally, they did an extensive medical exam. This included mental acuity testing. They told me they felt like, based on their vast experience, Sally might survive until the first part of June.

After receiving that news, it was very difficult to accept. Still, I also wanted my beautiful wife to be free of this awful plight. It was difficult to see her suffer any longer with this disease and the total confusion it caused for the patient. While I would be lost without her, my faith and trust in the Lord were strong, knowing all things were in His hands.

The report was shared with Johnna, Tonya, and Kenny. It also mentioned that the staff at Oasis Hospice had no explanation for her continued presence in her current condition. Because it was August, we were two months beyond when they thought she'd still be with us. Still, this gave me something to look forward to: her birthday and our upcoming anniversary.

We had always kidded each other about whether we would make it to 50 years of marriage or not. I always joked that Sally needed to behave better to make it to our 50th anniversary. But, in fact, it was more me needing to straighten up than her! She would always give me her special "look" and tell me not to worry about her. The message was loud and clear!

A few days later, I went to visit her after lunch, and she was still in the dining hall. The residents were listening to music and singing. "I love you, Sally," I said, seeing her big smile, sparkling eyes, and outstretched hands.

She said, "I know that. And I love you, too."

 **Glimpse:** When I looked at her, Sally gave me a big smile with sparkling eyes and responded, "I know that. I love you, too."

Next to her wheelchair, we listened to the music, and I sang along if I knew the lyrics. She was still very alert after the music ended, and we continued talking. Actually, most of the talking was done by me, while Sally only gave single-word replies.

But then she looked at me, placed her right hand on my arm, and said, "I'm going to be all right."

I kept looking at her, trying not to cry. Then she smiled and said, "I know you will be all right, too."

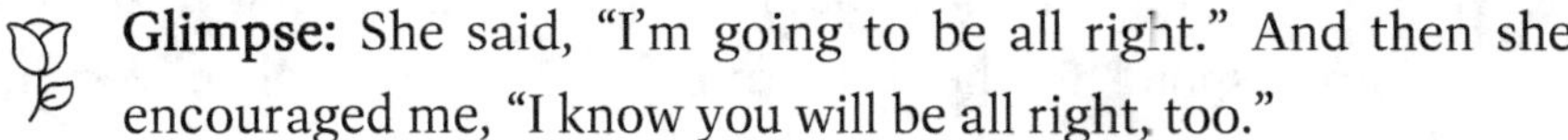 **Glimpse:** She said, "I'm going to be all right." And then she encouraged me, "I know you will be all right, too."

She then faded away, and her eyes became dull and lifeless, like a doll's eyes. I didn't know why this happened, but I'd learned to trust these brief messages through the glimpses of my beautiful wife.

The rest of the afternoon was spent with her in bed napping and me reading from the Bible to her, from one of her favorite books, The Book of Psalms. It was very enjoyable for me to read her the Bible, and it not only comforted her, but it did the same for me. The presence of the Lord was near, and I sensed Him speaking to us.

IT WAS LATE July, and Johnna was planning a visit for a long weekend. She would arrive on Thursday afternoon but would need to head back to Wichita on Tuesday morning. I was looking forward to this visit, and it was coming when Sally seemed to rally a little. When these brief periods happened, there was no way to know or understand why. Yet, they filled me and those present with such joy as we briefly experienced Sally's return to her true self.

During these times, Sally would talk in short sentences instead of just one word or a nod. Before this short rally, she was disconnected from everything. We had to realize that this is how dementia/Alzheimer's operates.

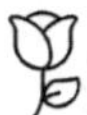 **Glimpse:** She rallied and would talk in short sentences instead of one-word answers or a nod.

LATE-STAGE ALZHEIMER'S (SEVERE)

Observations: In the late stage, individuals lose the ability to hold a conversation, respond to their environment, and control movement. They may still say words or phrases, yet have difficulty communicating pain. Personality changes occur, and they need extensive care. You may notice your loved one:

-Requires 24-hour assistance with personal care
-Loses awareness of experiences and surroundings
-Experiences changes in physical abilities, including walking, sitting, and eventually, swallowing

[cont'd next page]

-Struggles with communication

-Becomes vulnerable to infections, especially pneumonia

What You Can Do: The individual can continue to benefit from appropriate interaction, although they may not be able to initiate engagement. They may enjoy listening to music or receiving a gentle touch. Hospice may be beneficial to Alzheimer's patients and their families as it provides comfort and dignity for the end of life.

Gloria was a continuous presence in my life, as well as Sally's. Tears streamed down my face many times. Gloria would say the words and do the things needed to get me through that time of pain and suffering. I had worked to manage these feelings and was cautious not to have a breakdown in front of Sally, given that my upset would strongly affect her. Thus, it was vital for me to control these moments.

Sally was often asleep when I went to see her. During those times, I would sit by her bed, waiting for her to awaken. One time, a few weeks before Johnna's visit, Sally was asleep when I arrived. However, upon waking and seeing me, she smiled and dabbed my face. After asking if she would like to get out of bed and sit in her wheelchair, she responded with a gentle nod.

When pulling back the covers, I realized she didn't have any pajama bottoms on! This situation was very upsetting to me, and I went to find Aymie to inquire about my wife's partial lack of clothing in bed. Aymie allowed me to vent and then explained that they checked Sally's diaper every two hours. The aides could change her diaper more easily, and she'd stay asleep if she only wore a diaper. Wearing pants or PJ bottoms would cause her to wake up when they went to attend to her. While this was unsettling, it provided additional insight into my wife's treatment for this horrible disease.

THE DAY CAME for Johnna's arrival. She shared her navigation driving app so that I could track her journey on my phone during the five hundred-plus-mile drive. Her route from Wichita takes her through the Dallas metroplex. But thankfully, she made good time and wasn't delayed by heavy traffic.

Around 2:30 p.m. that afternoon, Johnna arrived at the nursing home. When she walked in, Sally was sitting up in her bed, awake and alert. Sally was 83 years of age, and she had been raised mainly by her strict grandparents as a child. Sally was taught to toss ripped jeans or convert them into shorts with pinking shears. One thing was for sure: you did not wear torn jeans out in public with holes in the legs!

But the trend now was for people to wear holey jeans with the worn threads showing. So, when Johnna walked into the room, her mother recognized her immediately and said, "Well, look who's here!"

They hugged and kissed, and Sally asked Johnna how she was doing. That is when Johnna moved back a couple of steps, and her mother spotted the jeans with holes in the legs. Her facial expression became one of concern, and she extended her hand and pointed at those holes in her jeans. Her hand shook a little, and she was visibly upset at Johnna for wearing such clothes in public.

Johnna started laughing and tried to convince her mother that these jeans were the style and "everyone" was wearing them. Her mother was not buying this line of reasoning.

Sally looked at me and plainly dictated, "Take your daughter and buy her some decent jeans. And do it now!" It was better for Johnna and me to leave Sally alone for her to calm down. Assuring Sally that we would be back in a little while with some decent jeans, Sally seemed to relax a little as we left.

Johnna and I chuckled over the recent events at the nursing home. Johnna explained that all the jeans she had brought were just like the ones she had on, so off to Walmart we headed to purchase two pairs of jeans without holes in them. Then we went to the house and placed them in the washing machine.

Sally was back to normal when we came back later. The new jeans Johnna wore caught her mother's eye right away. We saw her smile widen, and her eyes sparkled after she thanked me for taking our daughter on a shopping trip.

 **Glimpse:** Her eyes sparkled, and her smile widened.

During the remainder of our visit, Sally was very lucid. But around 8:00 p.m., she said she was worn out and wanted to rest. After getting ready for bed, we quietly left her to fall asleep.

The following day, Sally was still doing well, so we went outside to sit and watch the birds and admire the flowers. This outside area had knock-out rose bushes, which really looked more like small trees to me. The roses were small, about the size of a quarter, but they bloomed virtually all year long in Texas. Since Sally liked flowers, I'd often pick one and give it to her while we were outside. Each flower would be held with the utmost care, which would bring a lovely look to her face.

After a few minutes, I would place the flower she held into a buttonhole on her blouse or shirt, and that would make her so happy. She told us many times that the flower made her feel "special." We always told her she was special and that she was beautiful. But she felt otherwise, except in situations like this, when she wore a small rose on her buttonhole.

 **Glimpse:** Roses brought out Sally's inner beauty, and they gave her joy.

On Monday, we visited her in the morning. Then she retreated into her shell and did not talk at all. This upset Johnna, but I explained that this was just the way this brain disease caused her to be—up one minute and down for the next thirty minutes. At this time, we experienced more "doll eyes" than we did "sparkle eyes." The end was getting closer, and we knew it.

Johnna departed early the following morning for Wichita and mentioned needing to handle some financial matters upon her return. I told her to let me know if I could help, and she assured me she would. She also told me she just needed to work through some things. We shed a tear or two, and she headed for her home. The new jeans were left here so Johnna would not forget to wear them at her next visit and cause her mother to become upset.

A FEW WEEKS later, a text came over my phone from Johnna. It started with the words, "I hate to tell you this, but I have nowhere else to turn." Those are words a parent never wants to hear because we immediately know our child needs help. My first thought was, *why did you wait so long to come to me*? But, because it would make the person sharing the news feel even worse, I couldn't say it.

She shared that she was in a financial bind and might lose everything if she didn't get roughly $40,000. Johnna texted that she should've asked for our help sooner, though she thought she could manage the issue herself. She probably could have handled it then with just some consolation from us. But she had done it her way, and it did not work.

"Send me everything concerning your financial situation. This needs to include every weekly and monthly expense. I will talk to your mother and let you know later today what we can do to help."

She felt terrible about asking for help, especially knowing her Mom's expenses were so large. But she didn't have any other choice or know where else to turn.

Sally's mental state was usually at its weakest in the afternoons and evenings. But my first instinct was to do what we had done for over thirty years, and that was to talk to her about Johnna's current situation.

About thirty-five or more years ago, we had gotten ourselves in a real financial bind. Back then, we sat down together and came up with a sound plan to resolve the issue. It was based on Biblical principles and would help us become totally debt-free. We followed that plan for almost five hard years, but we were successful in accomplishing our goal. And, consequently, we had lived debt-free for nearly three decades.

As I sat next to Sally in her room, I explained that our daughter needed financial help once more. "What do you think we should do?" I asked while looking in her eyes.

She was obviously upset by this news, and tears welled up in her eyes. But she took me by the hand and said, "Can we help her?"

"It will be a challenge. But we can handle it."

The tears went away, and she smiled.

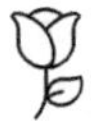 **Glimpse:** She smiled as only Sally could smile.

That evening, she said nothing more, but I felt she understood me.

Later, I called Johnna and explained that we would help her, on the condition that I make a plan for her to be debt-free before she retired in seven years. Isn't it funny that the Lord's perfect number of seven would come up in this life situation? It was His way of telling me it could be done, but we would need His assistance.

Johnna emailed a spreadsheet the next day, itemizing monthly debts and expenses. She had worked on this basically all night, but felt it was complete and accurate. After reviewing the information, she needed basically $22,000 immediately to take care of her credit card debt that had been negotiated down to this point. One credit card with a $10,000 balance remained for her to negotiate.

She provided her bank routing and account numbers so that we could send the money to her that day. The money would arrive in her account within a few days, allowing her to handle immediate needs without penalties.

Later that day, I went to our credit union and explained the situation to an officer. Wiring the money would be the best way, given the larger sum. The credit union officer contacted her bank and was given the additional information needed to complete a wire transaction.

Through the wonder of technology, Johnna received the money that same day. I told her to get those debts paid and send me copies of the checks and the invoices, which she did. Then, I began mapping out a plan using her spreadsheet, modeling it after the Financial Peace program and the 50-30-20 plan.

That plan teaches that we should use 50% of the *net* income for permanent bills, house payment, car payment, insurance, and the like. These are bills that occur every month and are a set amount. Then the 30% should be used for those bills that one gets monthly, such as electricity, natural gas, phone, and inconsistent bills, but the amounts vary from month to month. The final 20% should be applied to items like groceries, gasoline for your vehicle (in Johnna's case, diesel), hair appointments (crucial for a lady), and basically everything that doesn't fall in those other two categories.

The 20% rule means people must make sacrifices, a term disliked by many today. But this is where one must cut or reduce the frequency of extras, so the bills can be paid. Whenever you have money left over, which this plan provides when followed, it should be used to pay down debts by a fixed amount or eliminated completely.

Johnna agreed to implement that plan and went about paying off the negotiated credit card balances. We were on our way! She needed to give a bi-monthly account of her finances. I'd guide and support her until she changed her financial habits and was out of debt. By following this plan, she could retire on time. If she didn't, she could not retire and would have to keep working to eliminate her debt.

Grateful for our help, she stated she didn't know how she could ever repay the money to her mother and me. That wasn't our top concern at that point. She was reassured that life would bring along a need for us in the future, and she could help then. I told her not to even think about repayment until she was debt-free.

However, she needed to think of the money as a loan, not a gift. We did not want to enable her but help her get where everyone aspires to be: independent and debt-free.

We let her handle the matter on her own, but I checked in every month or two. And we continued supporting her in prayer as she worked out her plan to be relieved of financial burdens on her way toward retirement.

SEVENTEEN

September: Celebrations and Decisions

Loving you was one of the best decisions of my life.
ANONYMOUS

Seeptember came, and Sally started to slide downhill mentally and physically. Gloria increased her visits to three times weekly, and she advised that my wife's "final sleep" was near. The staff mentioned increased difficulty in feeding Sally as she really did not want to eat. Gloria said she'd come and try to feed her the next day at lunch.

September was Sally's birthday month. Also, it was the month we would celebrate our 50th wedding anniversary, if she were still with us. When the 16th arrived, I read her birthday cards aloud while sitting beside her wheelchair. Sally placed her hand on the cards and particularly enjoyed the cards with raised pictures on the front.

There were some raised blue Iris flowers on the front of the card I had chosen for her. She rubbed those embossed flowers, then looked up and smiled. After reading the verse on the card to her, I finished with, "Happy 84th birthday, my love."

"*Really* old!" were the only words she could utter.

"You're not really old. But you *are* on your way!" Sally smiled as she nodded her head. Even without words, we clearly understood one another at that moment.

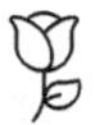 **Glimpse:** She smiled and said a few words, "*Really* old."

After reading the rest of her cards, she looked tired. "Are you ready to lie down and rest?" She nodded.

"Put your arms around my neck and hold on then," I said as she helped me lift her up and put her in bed. "Don't worry, I've got you," I confidently told her.

She helped me with the limited strength she had, and soon she was comfortably tucked into her bed and covered. An aide stopped by to check her, and she was fine.

WHAT CAUSES ALZHEIMER'S PATIENTS TO LOSE THEIR MOBILITY?

Cognitive decline affects motor control and coordination. Most Alzheimer's patients initially drag their feet without lifting them when walking. This results from muscle weakness and inflexibility in the hips. As the disease increases, muscle stiffness occurs and further impairs mobility.

Besides cognitive effects, the disease also brings about difficulties with spatial awareness and a loss of equilibrium. Vision problems also contribute to the patient taking shorter steps and being more prone to falls. Additionally, many of the medicines used to treat patients have a predominant side effect that causes dizziness.

OUR 50TH WEDDING anniversary was the following week, on September 23rd. Once again, I read her cards as she touched them and sensed them. When I read the one from me, she smiled, placed her hand on the front of the card, and looked into my eyes. Her eyes sparkled and were full of life, so I placed my hands gently on her cheeks and said, " Sally, we made it. We've been together for over 50 years—you and I—together. Can you believe it?"

She looked at me, smiled big, and then mouthed the word "Wow!" It was not audible because she hadn't been able to verbalize anything for the past two weeks. But I knew that she was excited to have made this milestone in our marriage.

Glimpse: Her eyes sparkled, she had a big smile, and mouthed the word, "Wow."

Gloria came to feed her that day. I had already left for a while to pull myself together and spend time in prayer and reading the Bible. A strong devotional time was the only way to get through these days. Every morning, I'd walk, cry, and ask God to send Jesus to take Sally home.

This was a really tough time for me personally, but it was obviously much worse for her—days of total confusion, not knowing what was happening, not able to communicate with us. It was difficult to imagine how Sally was dealing with this and how she really felt. She was no longer the vibrant woman I had known for over fifty years. Yet I had to encourage myself with my words to her: "We made it!"

Gloria texted me after feeding her and wanted to know how long it would take me to get to Focused Care because there was a decision to be made. Getting there would take around ten minutes, so I climbed into my truck and headed for the nursing home, wondering what decision there was to be made that day concerning my wife's future care. But, guessing was futile, so off I went.

Upon my arrival, Gloria was working at the table, using her computer to input data. She took my hand as I sat down next to her and explained that Sally's eating issues were because she could no longer swallow. She'd chew her food endlessly, then hold it in her cheek, unable to swallow. A scenario like this posed a major threat because if Sally were to gasp for breath while storing food in her mouth, she would aspirate and then need to be taken to the hospital for an emergency procedure.

Gloria told me my decision might be the toughest ever, and she'd support me. The decision was whether to stop feeding her or continue with the other risks involved in eating. Sally and I had already made plans years in advance—there would not be any feeding tubes or life support systems at the end of our lives, and that decision was recorded in writing as a living will. But by now making this decision, I was basically causing my wife to die from lack of food. I looked at Gloria and, in a calm voice, told her to stop all efforts to feed Sally.

On our 50th wedding anniversary, I had to decide not to feed my baby any longer. What a day. Talk about a high and a low! We had just celebrated fifty years together! On that day as well, I made the decision with a relative amount of certainty to no longer feed her.

The family was notified about my choice and the reasons behind it. Sally wouldn't live long now, perhaps two weeks at most. Gloria informed me that she and Sally's doctor decided on a low morphine dose for this period. This all took place on September 23, 2024, our 50th wedding anniversary. That night, I thought about how we had always wondered if we'd reach 50 years, and we did!

JOHNNA TEXTED ME to say that she'd be driving down on Tuesday with my sister, Martha. I was excited to see them both because this would be the first time seeing my sister in almost six months. Tuesday arrived, and Sally was doing well during our morning visit. She was reasonably alert and responsive with one-word answers, but that had become the norm— if she could speak at all.

My routine had been to assist her in brushing her teeth in the mornings, so that Tuesday morning I asked her if she would help me brush her teeth. She just gave me her little nod, telling me yes, so I pushed her wheelchair to her room and set up everything we would need to brush her teeth. Sally has an upper denture, which would have to be removed for the process.

The experience was always a challenge because she had to follow verbal directions and manipulate her mouth, both of which required mental and physical effort. For an Alzheimer's patient at her stage, this was definitely a challenge.

Though she was frail and unable to do much, she was able to take out her dentures for cleaning. She also followed the typical routine of using toothpaste and spitting out the residue. She did the same with the mouthwash. After everything was clean, she opened her mouth, allowing me to place her denture inside. All went well, and we celebrated this success with Sally getting a lollipop, something she really enjoyed.

It occurred to me that after over fifty years, we'd taken for granted simple daily routines that we typically handled ourselves. The once easy experience had exhausted her, so I took her back to bed. Now she slept almost constantly, and I knew her death was imminent.

JOHNNA AND MARTHA were on their way and would arrive that evening. It would probably be too late to see Sally, so we would visit her on Wednesday morning together. Around 8:30 p.m., they arrived, and I had already left Sally sleeping peacefully after my daily visit.

After they arrived, we had a light dinner and talked about the day and Sally's health. They asked a lot of questions.

One question concerned the morphine and how it was given to her. The medical staff placed the morphine, along with her anxiety medication, in a syringe, and then they just placed it inside her mouth next to her cheek. It was absorbed through her gums and the inside of her mouth. Johnna and Martha also asked if there was any prognosis as to how much longer she would live. However, there was no way of knowing exactly when, but it would not be long.

One indicator was that Sally's blood had started to "puddle," and there were places that appeared to be bruises but were in fact small pools of blood beneath the skin. A large, bowtie-shaped area of blood pooling was visible on her lower back above her hip. These places were not painful in any way to her, but they looked rather troubling. This pooling was just one sign that the end of her life on earth was coming. We then took time to pray together, asking the Lord to allow Sally's graduation from earthly life to heavenly life.

We went over my morning schedule so they would know what was going on if they couldn't find me. My sister was not known for her punctuality and needed a clear schedule. I would get up at 5:30 a.m., read my Bible and devotional, then eat a bowl of cereal. My morning walk came next, which was a little over three miles. After returning home, I shaved and showered, got dressed, and would be ready to leave at 8:30 a.m. for the nursing home.

Martha wanted a wake-up call, as she was unsure if she'd be ready by 8:30 a.m. Knowing early morning was the only time now when Sally would be responsive in any form, I would not miss any of that time. If Martha and Johnna were going with me to see Sally, they would need to be ready to leave at 8:30 a.m.

The next morning, I woke Martha, read my Bible and my devotional, ate my bowl of cereal, and headed for my walk. When I left for my walk, Martha was sitting at the kitchen table, drinking coffee and reading a magazine. Approximately one hour later, after returning, she was still sitting at the kitchen table. I went into my bathroom and shaved, showered, and got dressed for the day. Johnna was in the shower and was finishing up in the guest bathroom.

Right before leaving, my sister apologized. "I'm going to be late. Would you wait for me?"

"No, we need to leave at 8:30 to maximize Sally's period of alertness." Johnna was ready, so we headed out the door. Even with the early wake-up call, my sister was still getting ready and was left behind.

We arrived at the nursing home, entered through the front door, and spotted Gloria. "Sally has just had her medication and is resting. Text me if you need me for anything!"

"Thank you, Gloria." We headed for Sally's room.

When we walked in, Sally appeared to be sleeping. As was my routine, I went over, placed my hands on her pillow on each side of her head, leaned over, and said, "Sally, it's John, I'm here to be with you. I love you. Can I get a kiss?"

Waiting for a response, she puckered, allowing me to know she had heard me. And I would get my kiss, which would normally cause her to open her eyes. When she opened her eyes, I said, "Look who I found."

Sally turned her head slightly as I moved away and spotted Johnna. With a smile, she raised her hand to Johnna, which was a clear struggle. And she held Johnna's hand while our daughter spoke to her. The only response to Johnna's greeting was a simple nod, but that was enough.

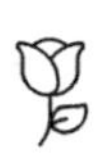

Glimpse: She would pucker, letting John know she heard him, and open her eyes. She then reached her hand out to Johnna and nodded.

She went back to sleep. We stayed until 1:00 p.m., when medication time came, and we knew she'd sleep until evening. As we were leaving, I texted Martha to ask if she was hungry. She was, so we went by and picked her up, and headed to the City Hall Cafe for lunch. She apologized for not being ready but asked how Sally was.

"She only had her eyes open for a short time and was responsive for about ten to fifteen minutes."

Martha was surprised at how brief her wakefulness was. "Do you think she will be awake later if we visit again after lunch?"

"She might open her eyes, though that is not something to expect as the day goes on."

We arrived at the nursing home after lunch and went to her room. I repeated the routine from that morning, but this time there was no response. Martha came up beside the bed and started talking softly to her, but there was no visible response. From what I have been told, even though we do not see any response, the patient hears you when you speak to them, but they may or may not respond. Sitting down beside her bed, I opened my Bible and read to her from the book of John, Chapter 14. I read to her for about an hour, with no response, but no sign of any discomfort either. She seemed at peace.

As we were preparing to go, Johnna inquired about staying with her mother for the night. We would have to get permission from Aymie, who quickly approved Johnna's stay for the night. We'd all head home, and Johnna could collect her things for her stay with her mom.

When we got to the house, Johnna asked if I had another Bible. I gave her one of her mother's, and then suggested that she look through it to see where Sally had written notes in the margins. Those scriptures were the ones she really liked. Johnna loaded up and headed back to the nursing home to spend the night with her mother.

THE NEXT MORNING, my routine was the same, and I again made sure my sister was awake. When I walked out of the bedroom dressed and ready to go, she was ready to go with me this time. She had learned how short the time with Sally was each day.

As we were leaving, Johnna pulled into the driveway. She said her mom slept well, but she didn't, so she'd shower and rest. We headed for the nursing home and went directly to her room. I leaned over her, placed my hands gently on her pillow, and said, "Sally, this is John. I am here to be with you. Can I get a kiss?"

She puckered her lips, and I was able to get a sweet, soft kiss. She opened her eyes and smiled. When I moved back, she spotted Martha and lifted her hand up toward her. Martha took her hand and started talking to her. Sally smiled, but then closed her eyes and went back to sleep.

Martha looked at me and made the statement, "Well, that was worth the trip! I'm glad I came."

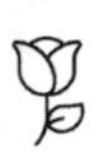 **Glimpse:** She would pucker, letting John know she heard him, and open her eyes. Sally then managed a smile and lifted her hand to Martha.

We remained there until around noon. I texted Johnna asking about lunch. She was awake and said she could eat. Martha and I went by the bakery and ordered three chicken salad sandwich combos to go. We retrieved our orders and headed home. My sister was astonished by the local bakery's delicious sandwiches, especially its famous chicken salad.

We got home, sat at the kitchen table, and gave thanks for the time with Sally and the meal. Then we discussed the current situation. Both Martha and Johnna had questions concerning Sally's end of life.

"What's going to happen next and when will it take place?"

"She's heading to a time, possibly within the next few days but no longer than one week, when she will enter what is called the 'final sleep.' Sally will be unresponsive to us once the final sleep process begins. The best we can hope for is a slight change in facial expression and maybe a small smile."

PREPARING FOR THE FINAL SLEEP

Observations: Personality changes occur, and they need extensive care. Physically, the body begins to shut down. One may notice:

-Blood begins to pool in parts of the body.

-They become less responsive to those around them; only slight changes in expressions occur until they become unresponsive.

-Morphine and other drugs are provided for comfort.

-They may assume a fetal position during the last hours/days.

What You Can Do: The individual may continue to benefit from the presence of loved ones, hearing soft words spoken or sung, and feeling gentle touches. Hospice may continue to provide guidance and comfort to the patient and the family during this time.

EIGHTEEN

The Final Sleep

Coming face-to-face with death brings clarity to
what's most important:
the extension of God's mercy to us and
our response of love to the Lord.

RAY NOAH

On October 1, when we arrived at the nursing home, I approached her bed, placed my hands on her pillow, and said, "Sally, it's John. I love you, and I am here with you. Can I get a kiss?"

She opened her eyes, and they were sparkling. She smiled and said, "Hi, baby, are you doing all right?"

"I'm all right." She then closed her eyes. "Are you going to rest?" She nodded.

I continued with these last words: "If Jesus comes and calls you by name, take his hand and go with him. I will be all right!"

She nodded again and went to sleep.

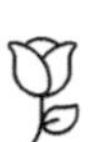 **Glimpse:** Sally opened her sparkling eyes, smiled, and spoke a complete sentence. "Hi, baby, are you doing all right?" She then nodded in response to John's words to her.

I did not realize that she would say nothing to anyone again, because this started the final sleep. It was a very joyous moment that Tuesday evening. I finished the evening with her by reading the Bible.

END-OF-LIFE RALLIES OR TERMINAL LUCIDITY

Terminal lucidity is when someone who previously lost the ability to communicate suddenly regains mental clarity. These unexpected episodes of lucidity are part of advanced dementia, and scientists do not fully understand what causes them. How long they last and what they involve differs among people. They may be fleeting or very dramatic. Typically, they occur within 24-48 hours of death and may include some of the following actions:

-Recognizing people around them
-Remembering who or where they are
-Recalling memories
-Asking for a favorite food
-Speaking in clear sentences
-Responding to questions
-Standing up and walking around

The caregiver should resist running to tell others, but be present for the patient and take advantage of the opportunity—it could be over within a few minutes. A rally is a wonderful gift; an opportunity to express how much you care for your loved one.

Johnna and Martha inquired about recognizing the final sleep. From what I had read and the information from Gloria, Sally would assume a certain posture normally resembling a fetal position. Once that happened, it would usually just be a few more days.

It was Saturday, October 5, 2024, and Johnna wanted to spend every night with her mother and would try to curl up in bed with her. She would not attend church with Martha and me the next day. Ready for worship, with my sermon, prayers, and announcements, I planned to check on Sally before going to church the next morning.

Martha asked, "What time will we leave on Sunday morning for church?"

"We need to leave at 8:00 a.m., which will place us at the church at about 8:50 a.m."

After opening the church and getting ready for the service, I knelt at the altar rail to pray. It would be great to have my sister with me that Sunday because Sally had always knelt with me. But she hadn't been able to be with me since the first of February.

My life had changed dramatically. While basically alone, I was spending as many hours a day as possible with my beautiful wife, partner, and best friend. That was what I lived for, and also for the precious memories of being by her bedside, though she seldom replied. Even though she could hear me, responding was a whole other story now.

When we were leaving for church, Johnna came home from the nursing home and told us that the night was totally uneventful. Her mother hadn't moved unless the aides came in and turned her. We hugged, and Martha and I left for the church in Leona. The worship service went well, and I informed the congregation that Sally was in her final sleep.

Soon, her battle with this terrible illness would end—it was difficult to say this about the person who meant the most to me. Sally had taught me about the life that the Lord had laid out for us and how to live it. She taught me how to love unconditionally, how to forgive, and how to be the man God meant me to be.

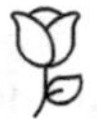 **Glimpse:** Sally's faith continued to influence John, even when she wasn't able to be in church with him.

After church, we stopped and picked up lunch for us to enjoy together at the nursing home. Sally's condition was unchanged, and the nursing staff's care continued. After eating in the dining room, we went to Sally's room and sat down around her. As usual, I reminded her, "I'm here with you. And will be here for a little while."

But there was no response. Sally's breathing was slow and shallow; it would not be much longer. I spent the late afternoon and evening reading the Bible to her.

Gloria, the hospice RN, stopped by for an unscheduled visit. We were worried at first, but Gloria's checkup ended with her telling us Sally was just in her final sleep and that she was fine. No one asked when she might leave this world because we really did not want to know. But in my heart, I knew it would be sooner rather than later.

Martha and I left Johnna there with her mother at 8:30 p.m. and headed home to get some rest. It had been a long day with the church service and being with my wife all afternoon. But I would have done nothing differently!

AROUND 3:00 A.M. I woke up. This was not typical for me and left me puzzled. But since there was no going back to sleep, I started to get ready. The moment I finished showering and getting dressed, Johnna knocked on my bedroom door. My heart sank, and a knot developed in my stomach. She told me that Sally was gone. She had left this world somewhere around 3:00–3:30 a.m. Martha woke up, and we informed her, and then we all convened in the living room.

Placing our arms around each other, we prayed. "Thank you, God, for taking Sally home to be with you forever. Please keep your arms around us during this time of great loss. In Jesus' name. Amen."

Johnna mentioned that a nurse from Oasis Hospice was already with Sally when she departed, so we headed for the nursing home. She was there at her computer, entering the information about Sally. Someone named Peggy was arranging the transport for Sally's trip from Huntsville to Memphis, Tennessee, and the MERI facility. There were other calls and arrangements to be made. But all of that could wait until I returned home.

As we entered Sally's room, there she was, lying motionless on her bed. She was on her back and seemed at peace. When her life ended, the muscles relaxed, and she was no longer in a fetal position.

I leaned in and told her I was happy her pain had ended and that she was with Jesus, giving her a gentle kiss. We couldn't help but notice that Sally was smiling. Not a big, huge smile, but a definite smile.

Glimpse: She had a slight smile on her face.

We held on to one another in silence and cried. But we were relieved that my beautiful wife's three years of suffering were over.

The RN from Oasis Hospice came by and told us she had heard from Peggy at Genesis, and the transport for Sally would be there in an hour or less. It wasn't long before Sally was on her way to Tennessee, her next resting place.

Martha was waiting for us at home. Johnna told us how she had been sleeping at the foot of her mom's bed and woke up just at 3:00 a.m. She presumed it was about time for her mom to receive her next dose of medication, so she had walked down the hall to the nurses' station and inquired about Sally's medication. The nurse would get it ready, but would first attend to Sally.

The nurse went to check on Sally, while Johnna went to the restroom. As Johnna came back to the nurses' station, the nurse was returning from seeing her mother. That was when she informed Johnna that her mother was gone.

Johnna reported that she neither heard from her mother nor felt any bed movement. Sally stopped breathing, and her heart stopped, and she went to be with God. Johnna found it hard to believe her mother died without a sound.

Based on her mother's words, I told her I thought she was prepared to go home with Jesus. She had made it to her 84th birthday! She had made it to our 50th wedding anniversary! And now she had made it home with Jesus and the angels!

NINETEEN

Genesis

The grave, the last sleep?
No, it is the last and final awakening.
Sir Walter Scott

Over twenty-five years ago, we had decided to donate our physical bodies to science so that we could help someone even after our physical death. Sally was always about helping others, and this was just another way for us to do that. So we made this decision together to continue to help. We had chosen to donate our organs to MERI (Medical Education and Research Institute), a place where young doctors use cadavers to practice surgical procedures.

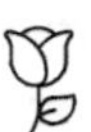 **Glimpse:** Sally always wanted to help others and did so even in death by donating her body to be used for training young doctors.

This opportunity allows doctors to use an actual body to practice knee replacements, hip replacements, spinal procedures, etc. The utmost respect is given to these cadavers because they realize what a gift that person has given them to hone their skills.

The morning of Sally's death, I called Peggy at Genesis, an organization that helps facilitate organ donations. Although expecting a voicemail, she answered on the third ring. She called me by name and told me that Sally would arrive there in about three hours. The Genesis team would remove the organs, and then Sally would be placed in her own cold storage facility.

Peggy would process all the necessary paperwork concerning Social Security and the State of Texas and would apply for her death certificate. This would occur that day, but the death certificate from Texas could take up to six weeks. She said that no one would mind the delay if I contacted people needing a death certificate before providing the official one.

Peggy continued. "Sally's body will remain at MERI up to one year, but no longer. Typically, it won't take that long. But we will let you know when her ashes are ready if you would like."

"Yes, please do!"

"Thank you so much for Sally's gift to MERI. Call me anytime with any questions you might have."

After that, I called Jennifer, my estate planning attorney, to let her know of Sally's passing and find out what to do. Peggy had already called, and everything was taken care of, she told me. After getting the official death certificate, I needed to go to the county to remove her name from the deed to our home.

Conversations with Peggy and Jennifer left me astonished at the seamless management of matters surrounding Sally's death. It also hit me that this three-year intense ordeal was over. The only thing remaining was to notify the entire family, which was done via group text messaging. I informed them that Johnna and Martha were with me and would stay a few days, leaving for home later that week.

ONE OF THE many things that we discussed together in preparation for our physical deaths was the celebration of life ceremony. We determined the ceremonies would be joyful, with music that wasn't somber hymns.

I had agreed to preside over Sally's Celebration of Life Ceremony at her request.

When a preacher leads a celebration of life service, the attendees should learn new things about the deceased. For any preacher, these services become personal even when they do not know or have any connection with the life they are celebrating. Yet, being the preacher in this situation and so close to Sally, it was a fight to keep the emotions together and not break down. All this said, I had promised her to be the one to perform her service. Some of my ministry friends thought it was a crazy thing to do, but they respected my decision. Two of them would be ready to take over for me if needed.

When considering the date for the service, I chose Saturday, October 26, 2024, as this gave me time to grieve. This date also gave me almost three weeks to prepare and helped me get mentally and emotionally ready. I had spent untold hours developing the service and considering what to say about her. The music had also been selected from songs Sally loved, and which had meaning to both of us.

Together, Johnna and I drove to Centerville, Texas, to Walters Funeral Directors, where we sat down with Aryn and reviewed Sally's celebration of life. When we arrived, Aryn greeted us, and I introduced her to my daughter. In the consultation room, I explained my expectations for the Walters team. Aryn knew me well, as I had officiated many services there for years. She had also been around Sally for almost 14 years.

The service would begin at 11:00 a.m., but the church would be open for visitors starting at 10:00 a.m. Parking availability at Leona Methodist led us to choose that location over Evans Chapel for the service.

The music choices and a copy of the service written in manuscript form were provided to Aryn for her team. She asked me who was going to officiate this service. Her reaction was puzzled after telling her I would do it, as she'd never witnessed a preacher husband lead his own wife's service. She wondered if I could get through it without breaking down, and we decided to have a "backup" pastor there just in case. Yet, I had promised Sally and planned to make every effort to uphold that promise and officiate her memorial.

Johnna asked her about putting pictures on a disk that could be viewed by all those attending. As long as the pictures were in their hands one week before the service, it would be no problem. Johnna would get the pictures to her digitally within a week, so there would be plenty of time to compile them.

After leaving the funeral home, we both felt very good about our scheduling of the service. Afterward, we visited the florist in Centerville to arrange the flowers for her service. We settled on a wreath with Sally's name on a ribbon across the wreath. The flowers would be several colors, but the base color would be red. Sally really loved red flowers. The time and date for the delivery were set, and we left.

All that was left was to set up a meal after the service for the family and a few close friends. We knew Jerry, the owner of The General Store, a restaurant in Leona. He would provide grilled chicken with roasted German potatoes, a vegetable, and a dessert shortly after the service, along with drinks.

Jerry inquired about who was officiating the service.

"I will lead the service," I told him.

"Do you think you can do that?" He was surprised.

"Well, I made a promise to Sally to do it, but Rev. Jim Jackson will be there to back me up if I cannot complete the service."

"That's a great idea!" he said.

We thanked Jerry for his help, then left for lunch at Pecan Grove, a small, family-run restaurant south of Leona. There were several local church members eating there who expressed their sympathy for the passing of Sally. They offered to help us with anything we might need. It was also an opportunity to share information about Sally's celebration of life service and where it would be held. Since I knew the General Store was open Saturday night, I asked them to speak to Jerry about assistance with the post-service meal. Then it was time to head back to Huntsville and prepare for all the family coming in for the service.

Johnna and I stopped by the house and dropped off some things. While we were there, my neighbor, Connie, came over.

"How are you doing, John?"

"As well as can be expected. We are making plans for a lot of family members who are coming in the night before Sally's service."

"Have you made any dinner plans for them on Friday evening, before the Saturday service?" she asked.

"We were hoping to include that after we booked the hotel rooms. Hopefully, the hotel will have a room large enough to accommodate thirty people for dinner."

"Well, find out the information and let me know where the dinner will be. The neighborhood golf group has discussed this, and we want to provide that dinner for you and your family."

What a blessing! If you've ever walked through grief, I hope that you have experienced this type of generosity and blessing from your friends. When things like this happen, and they are unexpected, it really touches your heart.

"Thank you so much for your help, Connie. You are a blessing. I'll get that information to you as soon as we know the details."

Johnna and I headed for the hotel, a brand-new Comfort Inn that had just opened nearby. This hotel was having its grand opening celebration! Since we needed to reserve a block of ten rooms, the lady at the front desk had never handled a reservation like that and requested the assistance of her manager, Karen.

Dealing with Karen was a genuine pleasure. After explaining our needs, she offered a special discount, as the event was a family gathering, the celebration of life for Sally. This helped us stay within the budget planned for the event. Karen needed the names and arrival times for each guest to make it easier for the desk attendant when they arrived.

Johnna and I started listing the names on a pad of paper to ensure we didn't forget anyone! Making a list was helpful because while working through it, we discovered we actually needed eleven rooms, not ten. I appreciated Johnna's help with the preparations, as my mind was clouded by grief. Thankfully, the hotel also had a room that was large enough to handle the family dinner. I texted Connie all the necessary information, mentioning Karen as the contact person to coordinate the setup.

About that time, someone from Focused Care called. They needed to meet with me to discuss the insurance payment concerning Sally. I must confess that my mind automatically went to the negative, having anticipated paying for expenses not covered by insurance. But when we arrived at Focused Care, we were invited to Jessica's office. My thought was, *Okay, now I'm sure I have a bill to pay!* Jessica accessed Sally's info, printed it, and presented it with an explanation.

Jessica told us she had never seen anything like this in her years dealing with insurance companies. But the insurance company had overpaid—yes, overpaid—Sally's claim. Because of this, a rather large refund would be sent in the next week or so. Another blessing! Remember the budget I had allowed for the rooms for the family coming to her service? This refund was going to more than cover those rooms, with a small sum left over.

Johnna and I were astonished. "Your mother is taking care of things for us!" I exclaimed. She smiled, and we thanked Jessica as we left her office. Surprisingly, the check for the refund arrived in less than a week— another shock, another blessing!

DURING THIS PERIOD of profound sorrow, many events were far from typical. Sally assured me, before she passed, that she'd organize and handle everything in heaven for me! I felt compelled to keep living as she'd shown me, to join her in heaven.

Psalm 91:11 (NLT) tells us, "For he will order his angels to protect you wherever you go." For me, it suggests that my angel, Sally, is still guarding and supporting me.

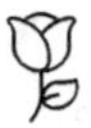 **Glimpse:** Sally was "organizing" things for the family from heaven. Blessings were pouring in.

Remember me telling you about the meeting Johnna and I had with Walters Funeral Home? When we left that day, Aryn told us she would be in touch concerning the cost of their service. Because I'd known them for over thirteen years and officiated at many of their funerals, I trusted these individuals.

Aryn called and explained that she spoke to the owners, and as she had requested, there would be no charge for Sally's memorial. When I passed this news on to Johnna, she said, "Mother is still working."

 **Glimpse:** Blessings continued to pour in.

Time seemed to fly, and the week of her service was here. Johnna returned on Wednesday to assist with final tasks. It was so good to see her. Over the years, we had our moments—normal things between a daughter and her dad—but we were so close now. She was a real blessing to me.

All the family members had responded and would be in Huntsville at the hotel before 6:00 p.m. that Friday night. We spent Wednesday and

Thursday just being together. We cooked and talked about the upcoming service.

"Are you planning on leading the service?" Johnna asked.

"Yes. I'm feeling confident about the service, and it would make your mother proud."

Friday came, and there were trips to the Houston airport to pick up relatives and get them checked into the hotel. After dropping them off, I asked Johnna, "Would you like to make a quick run by Dairy Queen?"

To which she replied, "That would be nice!"

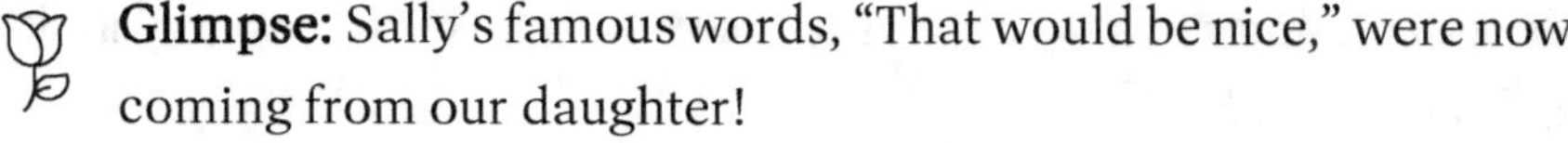 **Glimpse:** Sally's famous words, "That would be nice," were now coming from our daughter!

We sat there discussing how she loved ice cream and how she never needed any help to eat her cup. We also remembered that her cup was *her* cup. If you asked for a bite, she would look at you and say, "No!"

That might sound selfish (well, it actually *was* selfish), but considering the unselfishness of her life, it was just fine! We loved the way she would look at us and say, "No!"

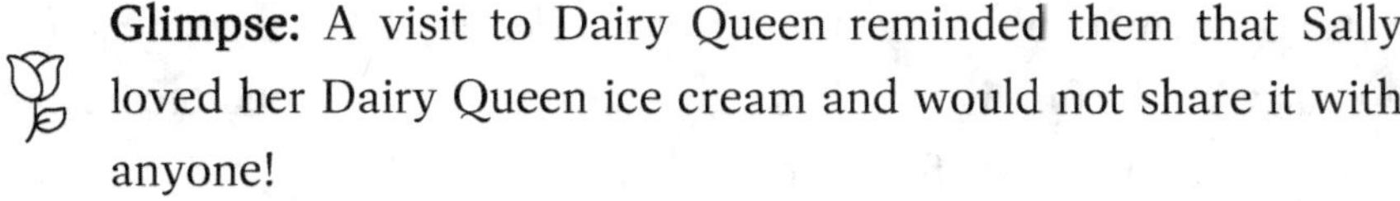 **Glimpse:** A visit to Dairy Queen reminded them that Sally loved her Dairy Queen ice cream and would not share it with anyone!

Connie had all the meal arrangements handled. The room was prepared, and the tables formed a large square to promote easy conversation. Guests could begin arriving around 6:00 p.m., and the food would be served at 7:00 p.m. The arrangements were perfect. The tables were set in a square, and black and white tablecloths had been arranged on them. I loved it, and Connie said the hotel manager, Karen, had arranged it all for us. Again, blessings just continued to come our way. These things might seem minor, but it felt like a fresh start after everything I'd experienced for three years.

Everyone had arrived and checked in, with a little extra time to freshen up before gathering for dinner. We were glad to meet, but we cried a bit, and shared stories and laughter about Sally's impact on us.

Dinner was set up buffet style. Once everyone was seated, I stood up and expressed gratitude for their presence, then offered a prayer of thanks for their safe arrival. Everyone ate and afterward seemed full and happy. It was nearly 8:30 p.m. before we headed home. Our friends' help made the evening run smoothly. And it seemed like we were being looked after from above!

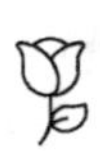 **Glimpse**: Touching memories of Sally's life, as told by friends and family, continued raining blessings down from above, with the impact she had on all she met. It felt like she was celebrating with us!

ON SATURDAY, I woke at about 5:30 a.m., which had become my typical wake-up time. After my Bible reading and prayers, I reviewed the service I wrote for my wife of fifty years. Johnna woke up, and we got ready for breakfast with the family at the hotel, because we knew we had to be back by 9:30 a.m. to get ready for the celebration of life.

It seemed like almost everyone was eating when we arrived. We prepared our plates, prayed with everyone, and then enjoyed this time together. Karen showed up and checked to see if everything was all right and if we were happy with what the hotel had done. She informed me she had taken care of late checkouts for anyone requiring them. Johnna and I headed back to the house, leaving maps for everyone with directions to the church.

We arrived at the church just before 10:00 a.m. I unlocked the church, turned on the air conditioning, and we joined together to pray. "Dear Lord, we ask for your help and continued blessings. Please give me the courage and strength to help me through the service. Allow me to honor you and make Sally proud. In Jesus' name. Amen."

Aryn's team arrived at 10:00 a.m. sharp to set up, which was completed in approximately 10 minutes. The florist arrived shortly afterward, from Centerville, with the wreath and a van full of flowers. Johnna determined the placement of the flowers after Aryn and her staff unloaded. The pictures of Sally were placed all over the chancel area, and flowers seemed to be everywhere. It was beautiful!

At about 10:25 a.m., many, many people started arriving. It was clear that the church, with a capacity of 120, would be completely full. Some of the church members began moving chairs from the family area and setting them up wherever there was room. Rev. Jim Jackson arrived, and he told me he was ready if needed. We settled on a single sign from me to him to tell him to take over. Jim and I went off together, and he prayed for me, asking the Lord to give me strength. Aryn had a copy of the order of service, which told her when to play each piece of music. We both agreed that I would signal when to begin and end the service's background music.

In the Chancel, sitting behind the pulpit, I was overcome with an unprecedented peace. I knew the Lord would give me strength, and I felt Sally smiling at me from her usual spot in the choir loft! Soon, Aryn turned off the gathering music, and the service, with approximately 155 people or more, was underway.

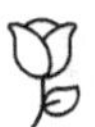 **Glimpse:** John felt Sally's sparkling smile from her usual spot in the choir loft as the service began. He continued the service

with unprecedented peace as he honored her life and the impact she had on others.

Epilogue

The heavenly distance between us now
does not change the power of our love.
MELVINA YOUNG

About seven months after Sally's death, I received a call from the Medical Education and Research Institute (MERI) concerning her cremation remains. Her stay there was complete, and she had served the young doctors well, giving them a human body to perform medical procedures on. They would be well-trained to help people when they were on their own after medical school. These young doctors learned how to do the procedures that would heal their patients, and in some cases, save lives because of their training at MERI.

They asked if I still wanted her remains. I immediately responded, "Yes!" After verifying my address, they confirmed the cremation remains would be shipped via express mail. They would arrive in one to three days. This was in the early part of Wednesday morning, and the remains were being shipped that morning. Most likely, they would arrive on Friday. This phone call and the fact that her remains would be in my possession in just a couple of days lifted my spirit tremendously.

The next day, I went to the postal facility in our community, opened my post office box, and found a card inside. Emotions began building within me as I approached the window to retrieve her remains. When I gave the card to the postal employee, she immediately retrieved the package containing Sally's cremation remains. Surprisingly, the markings on this package told everyone what the contents inside were. The postal employee looked at me and said, "May God bless you." After thanking her, I turned to head for the exit door with the package and said, "Baby, I've got you!"

When I arrived home, I took a few moments before opening the package. My emotions were still high, and there was a knot in my throat. I had learned during this journey that shedding tears was actually a welcome relief, so I never tried to hold those cleansing tears back—instead, I let them flow! Inside the package was the packing slip and a black sealed fiber container plainly marked. Now an urn was needed for her remains.

After searching online, I found the perfect urn for my baby's remains. After finding just the right one, the order was placed. A few days later, the urn arrived, and her ashes were placed inside. A special place was already set up for it, along with some favorite pictures of her, and the flag of the United States that was given to me by the people of Hospice. She now has her resting place, and I visit it frequently.

After I had received the call from MERI, received her ashes, and placed them in her special place, my life changed. My mental attitude perked up tremendously. This was a turning point. Now, over one year after Sally's graduation from this earthly life to her eternal life, things are as normal as this *new* life of mine will be for the immediate future.

Of course, from this point on, who knows what will transpire in my life, but I will trust that to my Lord. Currently, my life is as good as it can be, and once again, I can be happy.

As you have read this, I hope you have received some peace and comfort in your life as well. May God bless you on your path of healing as you move forward one day at a time. And may He bring light once again into your life.

Dementia may cloud memory and language, but it cannot sever a soul from the hand of God. With faith as your anchor, you can walk beside the one you love—praying, loving, and trusting the Lord to guide each step, even when the path grows unclear. And when the journey on this earth comes to its close, you can release them with peace, knowing God has already prepared the way and will carry them safely home.

Supplement

Sally's Celebration of Life

Words of Welcome

Jesus said to her, I am the resurrection, and [I am] the life. [Those] who believe in me, even though [they] die, yet shall [they] live, and whoever lives and believes in me shall never die," (John 11:25-26a, RSV [Emphasis Added]). *". . . I am the Alpha and Omega—the beginning and the end," . . ."the First and the Last. I died, [and behold] I am alive [forevermore]! And I hold the keys of [hell and death] . . .,"* (Revelation 1:8-18, NLT [Emphasis Added]). *"Because I live, you shall live also . . ."* (John 14:19b, NKJV).

Greeting: Friends, we have gathered here to praise God and to witness to our faith as we celebrate the life of Sally Burchell. We come together in grief, acknowledging our human loss. May God grant us grace and mercy, that in our pain we may find eventual comfort, in our sorrow hope, and in our death resurrection.

Our first piece of music today is "Nights in White Satin" by The Moody Blues.

Let me read from the Word of God found in Romans 8:26-30 (NLT): *And the Holy Spirit helps us in our weakness. For example, we don't know what God wants us to pray for. But the Holy Spirit prays for us with groanings that cannot be expressed in words. And the Father who knows all hearts knows what the Spirit is saying, for the Spirit pleads for us believers in harmony with God's own will. And we know that God causes everything to work together for the good of those who love God and are called according to his purpose for them. For*

God knew his people in advance, and he chose them to become like his Son, so that his Son would be the firstborn among many brothers and sisters. And having chosen them, he called them to come to him. And having called them, he gave them right standing with himself. And having given them right standing, he gave them his glory.

Please bow with me as I pray: Dear Lord, you are the one who formed us and gave us birth; you are always there to hear us pray, even though we sometimes are not ready to pray. You know what we need even before we ask, and you also know our fear in asking! Come here today and give to us your grace and peace, that as we shrink before the mystery of physical death and eternal life, let us see your light of eternity. Speak directly to each one of us the solemn message of physical death and life. Help us live our lives the same way those who know you and are prepared to physically die lived theirs. And when our days are complete, just as Sally's days are complete, enable us to physically die and be ready, like Sally, to go forth to eternal life. The life you give as a promise to all who accept you and your promise. In the Lord's name I pray. Amen.

Reading of the Obituary
Sally Jo Burchell
September 16, 1940 - October 7, 2024

Sally Jo Burchell was born on September 16, 1940, to Wilfred and Marjorie Smith in Wichita, Kansas. She grew up attending the Episcopal Church and continued to attend that church through her first marriage to Bobby Armstrong. During that time, she gave birth to a son, Kenny Armstrong, and a daughter, Johnna Armstrong. After the death of her husband Bobby Armstrong, because of a racing accident, she ran their business for over two years, and then she sold the business and the building.

On September 23, 1974, she married John Burchell, and Sally and John started a long life filled with many ups and downs, but always full of deep love for one another. Sally's father, mother, older brother John, granddaughter Kelsey, and a grandson, Paul, all preceded her in death. Sally is survived by her husband, John, her sister, Meg, and husband Rick Hayes, three children, Kenny and wife Robyn, Johnna, Tonya and husband Juan, Sister-in-law Martha Miller and husband Jake, sister-in-law Waunetta Walker, brother-in-law Mike Walker, eight grandchildren, and nine great-grandchildren.

Our second piece of music is "One Day at a Time" by Lynda Randall.

Reflection on Sally Burchell's Life (Rev. John Burchell)

When we look at our lives, we find something that is wonderful yet very complicated and complex.

If we were to look inside a really fine watch, like a precious Rolex, we would see all the wheels, gears, springs, brackets, and everything else inside that watch. We would wonder how all these things come together to make it work.

The same can be said about our lives. We start out as babies, grow into young children, mature into young adults, and go on to adulthood. And finally, we come to the end of our life here on earth in our earthen vessel.

When I look at all the things I have experienced in this life, I just have a problem seeing how it works or how it is supposed to work together.

But when I look at God's Word, I find in Romans 8:28b (NLT), *"God causes everything to work together for the good of those who love God . . .."*

When we look at the things that happen to us and around us, sometimes we find it perplexing how these happenings fit together, and how they will work together for good.

When we feel joy, sometimes we do not think too much about the happenings of life, but when we suffer the loss of someone we know and love, someone who has been a huge part of our life, we have a tendency to really take a hard look at what has happened.

Most of the time, we do not understand, and we seek comfort and understanding from friends and family. We want to know why, and we want to know why now.

We ask these questions because it hurts like no other hurt we have ever experienced. I cannot tell you how many times I have told people who have just lost a loved one that things will be "OK," well, I feel like I lied to them because I did not know the pain and the hurt they were suffering.

This is a difficult time for all of us who knew and loved Sally, and there will be no quick fixes.

This loss will never be replaced, but just like when we looked inside the fine watch, we could not understand how it all works together to give us the correct time, just as we have a problem understanding how good, peace, and joy will come from this loss.

But if we believe and trust in God, Jesus, and the Holy Spirit, great things will happen. Great things are on the horizon of our lives.

Life will be different. But through our faith and belief, we will once again experience joy in our lifetime!

This will happen because Sally is still here and a part of all of us. We have so many precious memories of her, and her relation to our life. We remember how she loved and affected each of our lives.

We are told in John 11:35 (NLT), *"Then Jesus wept."* Jesus wept, then and now, because he knows our pain and our loss.

In Romans 8:29a (NLT), we are told, *"For God knew his people in advance, ..."* God can look forward in time and know exactly what is going to happen.

God can look forward and know what decisions we will make in our lives, both good and bad.

We as humans do not have this ability. We can only look backwards and see what we have done and what has happened, not knowing what we will do in the future or what will happen in our lives in the future.

Each one of us will look back at our decisions and wonder if the decisions we made were the right ones to make. Yes, they were the right decisions because we made those decisions with the help of our Lord through prayer.

For all of us who knew Sally, we knew by the way she lived her life that she knew God. And we knew that she had a very intimate relationship with God.

In Romans 8:30 (NLT), we are told, *"And having chosen them, he called them to come to him. And having called them, he gave them right standing with himself. And having given them right standing, he gave them his glory."*

I remember one Friday morning not too long ago, when I told Sally that Jesus was with her, she looked at me and told me she wanted to go home!

I knew what she meant, and I told her that was where I wanted her to be!

When one of God's chosen goes home to be with their Lord and Savior, I know that God gives them all the glory in heaven.

They are placed in a place without pain, without troubles, without hardships, with complete memory, with nothing but glee and celebration. This is what we as believers in Christ Jesus are given by God the Father. Romans 8:31 (NLT) tells us, *"What shall we say about such wonderful things as these? If God is for us, who can ever be against us?"*

God loves us so much that he was willing to give his only Son so that we may enjoy eternal life in his presence. Today we are hurting, but Sally is smiling and laughing in the presence of her God.

Sally could go for a walk with her Lord in the cool of the day. All the questions that she wanted answers to, she has asked of God, and he has given her the answers.

The celebration of a life well lived here on earth has begun in heaven.

There can be no greater reward than to kneel in front of Christ Jesus and have him place his right hand on your shoulder, just like he did to Sally, and say, *"... 'Well done, my good and faithful servant...'"* (Matthew 25:21a, NLT). Amen.

Our third piece of music is "God on the Mountain" by Lynda Randall.

Let me read you this little poem, and then I will close in prayer.

"Miss Me But Let Me Go"

When I come to the end of my road
And the sun has set for me,
I want no rites in a gloom-filled room.
Why cry for a soul set free?

Miss me for a little while-but not for long,
And not with your head bowed low.
Remember the love we once shared
Miss me, but let me go.
When you are lonely and sick at heart
Go to friends we know.
And bury your sorrows
In doing deeds
Miss me-but let me go!
(Written by Christina Georgina Rossetti)

Let me close us with prayer: Eternal Lord, we praise you for the great company of all those who have finished their lives in faith and now rest from their life's labor. We praise you for all those dear to us whom we know in our hearts. We especially praise you for bringing Sally Burchell into our lives, and we know you have received her into your presence and presented her with the key to her mansion within your house. To all of us gathered here today, grant us your peace. Let your perpetual light shine on those you have received into your presence, and help us to believe what we have not seen. We pray your presence will lead us through our remaining years, and bring us at our physical end to be with them, and let us enjoy the joy of your home together. In Jesus' name I pray. Amen.

Our final piece of music is "On My Way, On My Own" by Lynda Randall.

About the Author

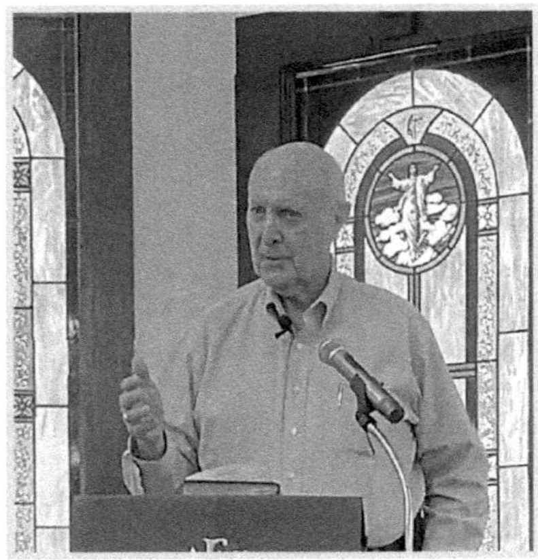

John Burchell hails from Wichita, Kansas. Shortly after his birth, his mother divorced his father. She remarried again four years later, with John being raised by his stepfather and mother in Wichita.

After attending public schools and graduating from West High School, he received an athletic scholarship to Wichita State University to play football. Following his college graduation, he went to work for a national auto manufacturer, where he managed a territory that spanned roughly one-third of Kansas.

While calling on one of his regular clients, he met his future wife, Sally, whose husband owned a high-performance auto repair business. Following her husband's unexpected death, Sally and John dated, fell in love, and eventually married. It was a marriage that lasted over fifty blissful years.

John's life completely changed after receiving Jesus Christ as his Lord and Savior. With his wife's and many supporters' help, he resigned from the auto business to commit himself to full-time ministry. He attended SMU's Perkins School of Theology and was appointed as a full-time pastor of a small Northeast Texas church.

John, an ordained Elder, continues his pastoral ministry even after retirement, assisting two small churches in central Texas. He has served these two churches for over fourteen years and plans to remain their pastor until 2031, God willing.

Outside of his writing and ministry work, John enjoys leading a local men's bible study and playing golf in his community just south of Huntsville, Texas. He and Sally successfully raised three children into adulthood. He has ten grandchildren, one of whom is in Heaven, and seven great-grandchildren.

You may contact John via email at: revjohnb11@yahoo.com